KILLER FISH

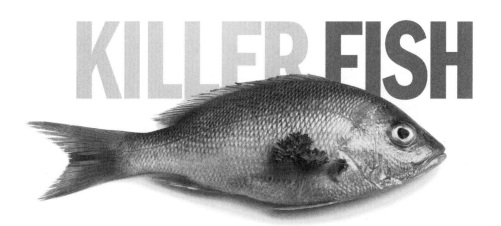

HOW EATING AQUATIC LIFE
ENDANGERS YOUR HEALTH

Brian R. Clement, PhD, NMD, LN
Director, Hippocrates Health Institute

· · · · · · · · · ·

HIPPOCRATES PUBLICATIONS
AN IMPRINT OF BOOK PUBLISHING COMPANY

Cover and interior design: Jim Scattaregia
Illustrations by Jim Barry

Hippocrates Publications, an imprint of Book Publishing Company
PO Box 99
Summertown, TN 38483
888-260-8458
bookpubco.com

ISBN: 978-1-57067-285-9

Printed in the United States

18 17 16 15 14 13 12   1 2 3 4 5 6 7 8 9

Library of Congress Cataloging-in-Publication Data

Clement, Brian R., 1951-
   Killer fish! : how eating aquatic life endangers your health / Brian R. Clement.
      p. cm.
   Includes bibliographical references and index.
   ISBN 978-1-57067-285-9 (pbk.) -- ISBN 978-1-57067-924-7 (e-book)
   1. Seafood--Health aspects. 2. Seafood--Toxicology. I. Title.

   RA602.F5C54 2012
   615.3'4--dc23
                              2012023356

Book Publishing Company is a member of Green Press Initiative. We chose to print this title on paper with 100% postconsumer recycled content, processed without chlorine, which saved the following natural resources:

· 38 trees
· 17,593 gallons of water
· 3,902 pounds of greenhouse gases
· 16 million BTU of energy
· 1,115 pounds of solid waste

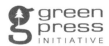

For more information on Green Press Initiative, visit greenpressinitiative.org.
Environmental impact estimates were made using the Environmental Defense Fund Paper Calculator, edf.org/papercalculator.

Contents

Foreword

More than forty years ago, I invited Brian Clement to join the Foundation Soleil in Geneva, Switzerland. My intention was for him to bring back to Europe the message that food is medicine, and he did just that. Along with his wife, Anna Maria Clement, he developed a state-of-the-art complementary health program at the renowned Hippocrates Health Institute. This extraordinary and transformative program should be used as a model worldwide, so that people everywhere can find more effective relief from the grip of disease, confusion, and melancholy.

Dr. Clement and his Hippocrates Life Transformation Program nurture people by teaching them to take total responsibility for their lifestyle choices. The program's comprehensive approach covers not only physical health but also emotional, mental, and spiritual well-being. It has been a great joy for me to watch the evolutionary progress of this program over the last several decades; the results that Dr. Clement and his team have achieved with tens of thousands of people are nothing short of remarkable.

One of the greatest illusions of our time is the belief that good health comes from elements outside ourselves, as demonstrated by our extensive use of chemicals, drugs, and vaccines. We have polluted our bodies and poisoned the global environment, creating an internal and external cesspool that separates us from the natural world and our natural state of health.

The human body functions brilliantly without the use of animal-based food. Fish, meat, dairy products, and eggs have no place in our diets. Factory farming and the manufacture of animal-based products have destroyed both our environment and our health. For millennia, natural healers, spiritual teachers, and shamans have taught the message "Do not kill." This universal tenet is receiving contemporary validation through current scientific research that proves poor health and environmental degradation are the result of breaking this fundamental code. It's time to allow all creatures, including fish, crustaceans, and other ocean dwellers, to live their lives fully, just as we aspire to live ours.

I am elated to present this landmark book, *Killer Fish*, which exposes the multitude of problems that come from the consumption of aquatic life and reveals how physical disease often manifests even when we eat foods generally considered to be healthful. If you believe that fish is a more nutritious choice than meat, go one step further and discover the whole story. Read this book and understand the delusion that food marketers have led you to believe. Not only will Dr. Clement convince you to stop consuming aquatic life, he will show you why plant-based diets are the only suitable fare for humans.

Killer Fish is a cornerstone contribution to the field of human health and has the potential to save millions of lives, both human and animal. Congratulations to you, dear reader, for having the wisdom to search for truth and apply it to your life. Enjoy peace, health, and joy with all that you do.

— **Christian Tal Schaller**, MD, author and pioneer
   in the field of alternative medicine and holistic health

What Do You Really Know About Fish?

C hances are, you or someone you know has fallen for the argument that fish offers a healthful alternative to red meat and dairy foods because of its omega-3 fatty acid content. But is aquatic life really safe to eat? If you think the answer is yes, be prepared for a rude awakening as you read this book. In these pages, you'll find startling evidence that you probably have not yet encountered.

The messages and information in this book could not have come at a more critical time: people the world over are eating more fish than ever before. According to the US Department of Agriculture (USDA), fish consumption in North America alone has increased by at least 50 percent since 1980.[1] Salmon, for one, has achieved newfound popularity because mainstream medicine has trumpeted praise for its omega-3 fatty acid content. Chapter 5 reveals why this praise is undeserved and will point you to the best sources of omega-3 fatty acids.

Authorities have known for some time that people who eat fish are putting their health at risk. An article in a December 2004 issue of the medical journal *Annals of Internal Medicine* stated: "But Americans have heard less about, and perhaps paid less attention to, various health warnings associated with fish consumption. Studies have linked overconsumption of certain fish (particularly popular ones such as swordfish, tuna steaks, Chilean sea bass, and some kinds of salmon) to neurologic deficits, cancer, autoimmune and endocrine disorders, and even some heart disease."[2] Chapter 2 introduces the human health risks related to fish consumption, chapter 3 highlights the dangers of eating raw fish and sushi, and chapter 4 describes how hormone-disrupting chemicals that are found in prescription drugs and personal care products are warping the reproductive life of fish and accumulating in humans.

The risks to human health are directly linked to the increasing contamination of fish and other aquatic species by industrial and consumer pollutants. This book shines the spotlight on many of these toxins, particularly mercury and polychlorinated biphenyls (PCBs). These and other dangerous substances are poisoning both wild and farmed fish, and anyone who eats fish also consumes these poisons. Chapter 1 describes the pollutants in fish and how their habitats have become tainted, and chapter 6 refutes the misconception that farmed fish are a safe choice.

You won't find much help from government agencies, or from the food and grocery industries either, in uncovering the health problems associated with fish consumption. While urging consumers to eat more salmon for its omega-3 fatty acid content, agencies such as the USDA and the US Food and Drug Administration (FDA) fail to sufficiently warn people that salmon contains high levels of PCBs and other toxins.

Nor do grocery stores place meaningful warning labels on fish that are known to harbor dangerous chemicals, leaving consumers blissfully ignorant of their health risks. When was the last time you saw a store post a prominent sign alerting consumers that tuna contains levels of mercury that are unsafe, especially for pregnant women? You've probably never seen such a sign, yet, as you will learn, the documented dangers of mercury contamination are a real and escalating threat to human health.

But human health is not all that is at risk. Chapters 7 and 8 focus on how human actions and fish consumption threaten environmental health. In fact, some experts predict that sea life will perish in our lifetime.

No book about the killing and eating of aquatic animals would be complete without a discussion of the ethical aspects of human conduct and cruelty toward other life forms. There is not only the question of cruel treatment, though that is justification enough to refuse to participate in the business of animal agriculture. In addition, there exists a whole other dimension to consider, which is the extent to which an animal's intelligence should determine its use as a food source. The smarter and more socially advanced the life form is relative to human intelligence, the argument goes, the less likely it is to be served at the dinner table.

For example, unless you live in China or Southeast Asia, or unless you were starving, you probably haven't considered eating a dog, because that species is viewed as an intelligent and useful human companion in most parts of the world. However, some people who refuse to eat land creatures in recognition of their social versatility and ability to reason, or the cruelty inflicted while raising them, don't think twice about eating or mistreating fish. It's as though these creatures are too lowly to warrant compassion.

Scientific research affirms that fish are highly evolved creatures. In his thought-provoking book *Eating Animals,* Jonathan Safran Foer points out that since the 1990s, more than five hundred published papers have dramatically expanded our knowledge about the surprising sophistication of fish intelligence. "Fish build complex nests, form monogamous relationships, hunt cooperatively with other species, and use tools," Foer writes. "They recognize one another as individuals (and keep track of who is to be trusted and who is not). They make decisions individually, monitor social prestige, and vie for better positions. (To quote from the peer-reviewed journal *Fish and Fisheries:* they use 'Machiavellian strategies of manipulation, punishment, and reconciliation.') They have significant long-term memories, are skilled in passing knowledge to one another through social networks, and can also pass on information generationally. They even have what the scientific literature calls 'long-standing cultural traditions for particular pathways to feeding, schooling, resting, or mating sites.'"[3]

People who care about the well-being of animals, including fish, are also more inclined to care about the well-being of other human beings. History will judge our culture for how civilized and humane we have been in our treatment of all life forms. As you read this book and absorb its message, please keep in mind that your eating habits and buying decisions help determine not only your own health but also the fate of entire species and the ecosystems on which they depend. Our awareness can constantly motivate us to change our actions and, ultimately, change the human relationship to food, nutrition, and the planet's ecological health . . . one bite at a time.

KILLER FISH

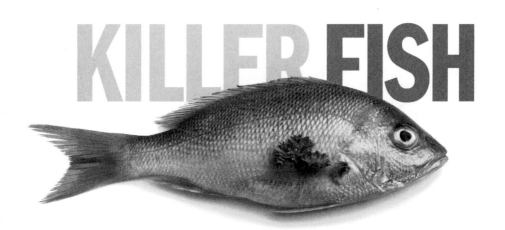

HOW EATING AQUATIC LIFE
ENDANGERS YOUR HEALTH

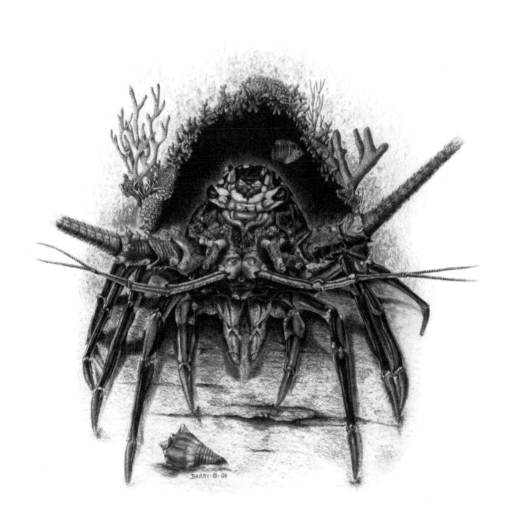

CHAPTER ONE

How Aquatic Life
Got Contaminated

It's about time that people who are concerned about their own health and the health of the planet become familiar with three terms coined by *Chasing Molecules* author Elizabeth Grossman: fliers, swimmers, and hoppers.[1] This terminology may sound like a list of options for a frequent traveler program, and in a strange way, that's exactly what it is, except these travelers aren't human.

The travelers in this case are molecules of toxic substances produced by industry and commerce. While invisible to the naked eye, these fliers, swimmers, and hoppers take up residence inside all life forms, including humans, and many of them are virtually immortal and practically indestructible. Being highly mobile and uncontainable, they can pop up anywhere on the planet, having traveled thousands of miles for months or even years before finally finding a "home" inside of fish and, eventually, inside of you.

These hitchhiking contaminants range from pesticides, fungicides, and herbicides to heavy metals (mercury being the most common), flame retardants (especially those called PBDEs), water- and stain-repellant chemicals (known collectively as PFCs), and numerous other industrial compounds. These molecules fly, swim, and hop about with the greatest of ease on wind and water currents. (For more information about these toxins, see sidebar, page 3.)

Persistent organic pollutants (POPs) are a principal category of world travelers that take refuge inside of human and aquatic life. They include the pesticide DDT, polychlorinated biphenyls (PCBs), and dioxins. The United Nations Environment Programme has stated: "Exposure to persistent organic pollutants can lead to serious health effects, including certain cancers, birth defects, dysfunctional immune and reproductive systems, greater susceptibility to disease, and even diminished intelligence."[2]

Fliers travel primarily by air, attached to dust particles on the wind or in storm systems. Swimmers are mostly restricted to oceans and other bodies of water. Propelled by wind and water, contaminants that originated in North America can end up in Europe, and pollutants generated in China can travel to the United States. In fact, molecules that hitchhike on dust particles can make the journey from China to California in just a few days.

Some hitchhikers are versatile and jump from air to water and sometimes back again. These hoppers can morph into a gas, liquid, or particle.[3] Changes in form are influenced by various factors, such as chemical structures, temperature fluctuations, and atmospheric conditions. Rain and snow are ideal carriers, depositing hoppers in oceans, lakes, and rivers, where they are absorbed by aquatic life.

Because toxins easily cross-pollute between regions of the world, and because many of them persist in the environment for decades or more after being released, any one nation's attempt to put the genie back in the bottle is an ultimately fruitless endeavor. Limiting toxic emissions within a country's borders does not protect it from toxins created elsewhere. And the number of contaminants is always increasing. New chemical hoppers are constantly being created in laboratories and added to industrial processes and consumer products.

Meet Fliers, Swimmers, and Hoppers

Our world is home to many toxic hitchhiking molecules. Here is more information about these ubiquitous travelers:

- **Pesticides, fungicides, and herbicides.** This broad category of pollutants includes aldrin, chlordane, dichlorodiphenyldichloroethane (DDD), dichloro-diphenyltrichloroethylene (DDE), dichlorodiphenyl-trichloroethane (DDT), dieldrin, endrin, heptachlor, hexachlorobenzene (HCB), hexachlorocyclohexane (HCH), and toxaphene. Many of these substances have been banned in the United States and other parts of the world for decades, yet they persist in the environment.

- **Heavy metals.** Mercury is the most common heavy metal contaminant found in fish and other aquatic creatures. The term methylmercury refers to the various toxic compounds of mercury that accumulate in living organisms.

- **Flame retardants.** These toxic and persistent molecules are used in the manufacture of textiles, plastics, and other products. They include polybrominated diphenyl ethers (PBDEs).

- **Water- and stain-repellant chemicals.** These chemicals are known collectively as perfluorinated compounds (PFCs). They can be found in the slick paper coating used on microwave popcorn bags and pizza boxes. Two well-known brand names are Teflon and Gore-Tex.

The contaminants found in aquatic environments have a real and growing effect not only on fish and other sea creatures but also on humans. These chemicals love fat, meaning that once they are absorbed by fish and other creatures, they bioaccumulate in fat cells. Simply put, they establish a mobile home park and invite all of their "friends" over to hang out. Bioaccumulation also happens when humans eat fish and animal flesh that is tainted with these chemicals. The toxic tourists settle into the fat cells of their human hosts for a long visit and, in the process, create a lot of mischief (see chapter 2).

How Bad Is It? Let's Start with Mercury

You've probably heard a lot about high levels of mercury being found in tuna, a saltwater fish. But are you aware that this heavy metal is also found in freshwater species of fish?

You wouldn't have learned about the widespread contamination of freshwater fish by following mainstream media reports. Nor would you have learned that the primary source of mercury contamination, as well as other types of contamination in both freshwater and saltwater species, is our own industrial civilization.

Naysayers within the scientific and industrial communities have long contended that most of the mercury being detected in fish and aquatic sediments comes from natural geologic leaching. However, numerous studies conducted over the past decade have shown that this argument no longer carries any weight. Much of the mercury we are seeing in fish comes from industrial pollution. When mercury by-products enter water, whether freshwater or salt water, they are converted into methylmercury, which is easily absorbed by fish. The methylmercury bioaccumulates up the food chain through predator fish until it's absorbed by humans. The only way to avoid contamination by these forms of methylmercury is to avoid eating fish.

The following series of studies document that mercury contamination is the result of the atmospheric spread of mercury from human sources. In a 2007 article in *Environmental Science & Technology*, researchers reached this conclusion: "Our findings suggest that atmospheric transport is a key factor relative to Hg [mercury] in fish across the western United States."[4] The researchers collected and analyzed 2,707 large fish from 626 streams and rivers across twelve western US states and discovered that mercury concentrations were high in all of the fish they sampled.

The previous year, two scientists from the Woods Hole Oceanographic Institution published a study in the same journal that evaluated concentrations of methylmercury in freshwater fish from every state. They reported, "The accumulation of MeHg [methylmercury] in wild fish populations is linked to atmospheric Hg [mercury] loadings, two-thirds of which are estimated to be from anthropogenic sources."[5] Anthropogenic is a term that refers to the influence of human beings on nature.

Even earlier than this, four marine scientists from various universities reported similar findings: "There is a broad and geochemically consistent database indicating that, over large regions of the globe, human-related Hg [mercury] emissions have increased relative to natural sources since the onset of the industrial period."[6] This should end the previously contentious debate about whether naturally occurring sources of mercury in the environment or human-generated sources are the principal culprits in contaminating aquatic life and, consequently, endangering human health.

In the United States, the Great Lakes and California waterways are particularly plagued by mercury contamination. The Great Lakes, the largest surface body of freshwater on the planet, are a major receptacle for industrial pollutants. From the 1970s to 2007, long-term monitoring data documented an escalation in mercury levels in several fish species in the Great Lakes. Lake Erie walleye, for example, continue to show increasing levels of mercury contamination. Mercury levels in this species have remained steady in Lake Ontario for two decades, while levels have increased over the past ten years in Lake Erie.[7]

A 2004 report by the California Department of Health Services warned about mercury contamination and the health risks associated with consuming fish from the entire Sacramento-San Joaquin River Delta and all of its tributaries in the northern part of the state. According to the report, "Mercury concentrations in several species of fish exceed the health-based screening values set by the US Environmental Protection Agency."[8]

In the San Francisco Bay, all of the fish species carry unsafe levels of mercury. This is a result of gold mining, which started with the California gold rush of 1849. Mercury was used to amalgamate the gold at slurry mines in the Sierra Nevada Mountains. Nearby streams carried the mercury waste into delta waterways, and it eventually washed into the San Francisco Bay. The contamination is so thorough that there is no hope of ever completely cleaning it up.

Mercury levels in striped bass, sturgeon, and shark, in particular, are so high in the San Francisco Bay and related waterways that the California Office of Environmental Health Hazard Assessment has issued health warnings that women of childbearing age or pregnant women and children should eat no more than one meal that includes these fish each month.[9] Women beyond childbearing age and men should consume no more than two of these fish meals each month.

My advice, as you can imagine, is not to eat any of these fish. I don't believe consuming any level of mercury is safe for long-term health. The government does not agree. In 1969 the US Food and Drug Administration (FDA) established 0.5 parts per million (ppm) as the maximum safe level of mercury contamination in fish.

In 1979 that level was arbitrarily raised to 1 ppm, despite the well-documented neurological problems in humans caused by mercury exposure. (Parts per million is a measure of the number of chemical molecules; one part per million is roughly equivalent to about one milligram per liter of water.)

Let's consider an example that was calculated using the average level of mercury contamination for chunk white canned tuna. A normal child weighing forty-five pounds who eats six ounces (about one can) of chunk white tuna has ingested *four times* the recommended level of mercury.

Table 1 lists the maximum mercury concentration levels in the most contaminated types of fish. This information is based on data compiled by the FDA from various scientific studies conducted over three decades.

Table 1. Mercury levels in fish

Type of fish	Maximum measured mercury level (in parts per million)
Shark	4.5
Tilefish (from Gulf of Mexico)	3.7
Swordfish	3.2
Chilean sea bass	2.1
Tuna (fresh or frozen)	1.8
King mackerel	1.6
Halibut	1.5
Tuna (yellowfin)	1.4
Bluefish	1.4
Snapper	1.3
Grouper	1.2
Orange roughy	1.1

Source: US Food and Drug Administration[10]

Pesticides, PCBs, and Dioxins

There has never been any debate about the source of certain categories of contaminants in fish, such as the whole family of dioxins, PCBs, and pesticides. All are clearly and widely seen as by-products of industrial processes.

Just as many scientific studies have demonstrated the dangerous levels of mercury in fish, additional research from all over the world has documented the presence of other contaminants, either alone or in conjunction with mercury. For example, a study was done to determine the concentrations of environmental toxins in fish eaten by the Ojibwa tribe in the Upper Great Lakes region. Researchers found PCBs and seventeen other organochlorine compounds in lake trout, whitefish, and walleye. Lake trout and whitefish from Lakes Michigan and Huron had the highest concentrations of organochlorines, whereas mercury, at 0.58 parts per million, was highest in walleye. PCBs were found in all lake fish sampled.[11]

To illustrate how persistent and virtually indestructible some of these contaminants continue to be, we need only look at the continuing presence of the insecticide toxaphene in the sediments of the Great Lakes. Banned for all uses in the United States in 1986 because it is highly carcinogenic, toxaphene had been used widely on cotton and soybean crops in the midwestern United States. Toxaphene was also frequently used in lakes to kill unwanted fish species. Certain fish, such as salmon, store the chemical in their fat much more readily than other animal species, possibly because toxaphene was manufactured to be used in water.

When sediment cores from Lakes Superior, Michigan, and Ontario were analyzed, toxaphene was detected in alarming levels, demonstrating how slowly it degrades. Once absorbed by fish, it can biomagnify up the food chain. Researchers determined that the continuing buildup of toxaphene in sediment and aquatic life was caused by atmospheric sources. The chemical originated far away but traveled on air currents, probably attached to dust particles, before ending up in the lakes.[12]

Fish in the lakes and streams of California are also affected by pollutants. You may have heard of the Donner Party, the nineteenth-century wagon-train pioneers who were trapped in California's Sierra Nevada mountain range in a winter snowstorm and resorted to cannibalism to survive. Donner Lake was named for them to mark the area of their encampment. It is locaterd alongside Interstate 80 between Sacramento, California, and Reno, Nevada.

The fish in Donner Lake have mostly become unfit for human consumption as a result of PCB and mercury contamination. California's Office of Environmental Health Hazard Assessment issued a permanent fish advisory for the lake on January 27, 2011. The warning stated that fish samples caught in the lake contained detectable levels of mercury, PCBs, and a few other chemicals and that people should drastically cut back their consumption of brown trout and lake trout.[13]

A series of studies done between 1999 and 2002 found that the waters of Canada's Arctic and subarctic regions were so highly polluted with mercury that fish species such as lake trout, pike, and walleye carried mercury levels exceeding government safety standards. "New research on PDBEs and perfluorinated compounds determined that these contaminants are widespread in freshwater fish and concentrations may be increasing," concluded a Canadian team of scientists in 2005. "Global warming is a major issue of concern for Arctic and subarctic waters and may have adverse impacts on contaminant levels in fish."[14]

In 2010 scientists analyzed nine fish species that were caught in waters off the Aleutian Islands of Alaska. They discovered that the fish were carrying significant concentrations of POPs, including PCBs and three pesticides (DDE, mirex, and HCB). The highest level of DDE, a breakdown component of the insecticide

DDT, was found in sockeye salmon, while the highest PCB level was found in rock sole. The researchers stated: "All species [of fish studied] would trigger strict advisories of [no more than] between two and six meals per year." Furthermore, the scientists noted that their results raise questions about whether these fish are safe to eat at all.[15]

In Japan, researchers conducted blood tests on 131 men and 122 women (ages twenty to seventy-six) who lived along the coast. They measured levels of PCBs and dioxins, such as PCDDs. Study participants completed a dietary questionnaire that the researchers used to determine both the amount and types of fish commonly consumed. Plasma concentrations of a biomarker of fish intake were positively associated with blood levels of dioxins. The researchers stated: "The frequency of intake of coastal fish, such as horse mackerel, mackerel, and sardine, was associated with concentrations of PCDFs and PCBs. The intake of raw fish was positively related to total dioxins and PCBs."[16]

As part of a 2005 study in Singapore, scientists measured the levels of several heavy metals and POPs in the edible portions of twenty types of commonly consumed seafoods, such as gray prawns, eel, and salmon. They found that the insecticides chlordane and DDT, in addition to PCBs, were the primary contaminants, with the highest concentrations found in salmon fillets and green mussels. The authors discussed these contaminants and related cancer risks in their conclusion: "Daily intake of DDTs, heptachlor, and PCBs in seafood exceeded the conservative cancer benchmark concentrations set by the US Environmental Protection Agency, suggesting that a significant number of people are potentially at risk in Singapore over a lifetime from seafood consumption."[17]

In 2001 a team of toxicologists collected samples of eleven fish species caught in Europe's largest wetland, the Danube Delta in Romania. They measured concentrations of PCBs, PBDEs, and organochlorine pesticides (such as DDT, HCH, and HCB) in the fish and water sediments. DDT was the predominant pollutant in all samples and was found in both fish muscle and liver. The next highest concentrations were of PCBs.[18]

Between March and June of 2006, a group of toxicologists acquired food samples from twelve cities in the Catalonia region of northeastern Spain. They measured concentrations of PBDEs in this wide variety of foodstuffs. By far the highest concentration of total PBDEs turned up in fish and shellfish, at levels nearly twice that of the next most contaminated category of foodstuffs, oils and fats.[19]

Table 2. Common contaminants in fish

Toxin	Type	Effects	Fish with high levels
Dichlorodiphenyltrichloroethane (DDT)	insecticide	endocrine disruption, diabetes, and possibly cancer	sockeye salmon
Hexachlorobenzene (HCB)	fungicide	neurological problems, enlarged thyroid and liver	wild salmon, mackerel
Polychlorinated biphenyls (PCBs)	industrial chemical used as coolant fluid	endocrine disruption, neurological problems	black bass, carp, channel catfish, largemouth bass, and smallmouth bass
Polycyclic aromatic hydrocarbons (PAHs)	by-products of burning fuels	DNA damage, cancer, and lower IQ	Atlantic mackerel, Atlantic salmon, blue whiting, clams, herring (smoked), mussels, rainbow trout (farmed), and shrimp

Sources: [20, 21, 22, 23, 24, 25, 26, 27, 28, 29, 30]

Check Your State's Fish Advisories

Most states periodically post advisories, usually on a website, that warn consumers about fish species that pose a risk to human health if eaten. A state agency such as the Department of Health is typically in charge of issuing advisories about the fish caught in its home state.

Have you ever checked the warnings posted by your state? Probably not. Few consumers even know about these advisories, much less use them to guide their buying and eating decisions. Yet paying attention could protect your health, if not your life.

In my own state of Florida, the Department of Health issues fish consumption advisories in cooperation with the state Department of Environmental Protection and the Fish and Wildlife Conservation Commission. Let's take a look at what was posted on the Florida Department of Health website in 2011.[31]

After first proclaiming that eating fish is an important part of a healthful diet, the state agency posts twenty-eight pages of single-spaced warnings about species of fish that inhabit dozens of rivers, creeks, canals, lakes, and coastal waters. In total, **Do Not Eat** warnings (in bold capital letters) are issued for various species in ninety-seven bodies of water. Several hundred additional listings warn consumers not to eat some types of fish more than once a month if they want to avoid health consequences.

Here are just a few examples of the **Do Not Eat** warnings:

- Hunters Lake, Hernando County: largemouth bass and black crappie
- Lake Annie, Highlands County: largemouth bass, bowfin, and gar
- All coastal waters: blackfin tuna and king mackerel

The website also lists some of the contaminants, including dioxins, PCBs, pesticides, and saxitoxin, detected in catfish and other fish species. Given the documented dangers of eating fish, the state agency's claim that fish are an important part of the human diet seems designed to protect the fish industry and the state's economy rather than human health.

North American Fish Advisories

The US Environmental Protection Agency (EPA) maintains a website that posts fish advisories—which are basically fish contamination alerts to consumers—that have been published by agencies of the fifty states, the four US territories, and all of Canada's twelve provinces and territories. To find this information, go to water.epa.gov and search for "fish consumption advisories."

Some Things to Keep in Mind

It's easy to lose sight of how widespread the contamination of aquatic life has become and the potential effects on human and planetary health. Keep in mind that the toxins listed in this chapter include just the handful of chemicals that fish have been tested for so far, which means that numerous other toxins may be present in fish tissue. We also have not yet explored the emergence of "gender-bender" fish that are affected by the many endocrine-disrupting chemicals that pollute the world's waterways (see chapter 4).

A second thing to remain aware of is the process of biomagnification. For example, mercury levels accumulate over time, so older and larger fish, such as swordfish and sharks, carry around abundant toxins that they absorb from eating smaller sea animals, such as krill and shrimp. An April 2007 article in *National Geographic* quantifies the effect: "Fish at the top of the food chain can contain mercury levels that are 10,000 to 100,000 times higher than those of their environments."[32] The same principle holds true for many other hopping toxic chemicals. They biomagnify up the food chain, hiding in fat cells until they are consumed and then released into more complex life forms, such as human beings.

Also of concern are the long-term effects of environmental disasters. For example, marine scientists monitoring schools of migratory fish off the coast of California have discovered that blue-fin tuna are contaminated with radioactivity. The source was leakage from the nuclear power plant that was damaged during the March 2011 earthquake and tsunami in Japan.[33] Amounts of radioactive cesium (an elemental metal) in the fish were ten times higher than amounts measured in the same species prior to the nuclear plant disaster. The new levels surprised scientists because it had been theorized that fish could metabolize radioactive substances. This finding should be of particular concern to sushi eaters since Pacific bluefin tuna is offered as a prized delicacy in sushi restaurants.[34]

The second disturbing development has emerged more than two years after the BP oil spill in the Gulf of Mexico, where the environmental damage can still be seen in the form of diseased fish and other aquatic life. A team of scientists sampled fish in both shallow and deep waters stretching from Florida to Louisiana. They found widespread evidence that the oil spill and the chemical dispersants used in response have seriously damaged up to 10 percent of some fish types, causing immune system impairment, genetic abnormalities, physical deformities, and liver and lung disease.[35]

Lastly, there is the question of additive, or synergistic, effects that occur when multiple chemical toxins are absorbed from marine life and other sources. Toxins interact to multiply each other's effects. Few studies have been done to document these unpredictable and highly dangerous effects, yet we know synergy is a principle of nature. Risks continue to escalate for both marine life and humans as the number of toxins and their concentration levels in our environment increase over time.

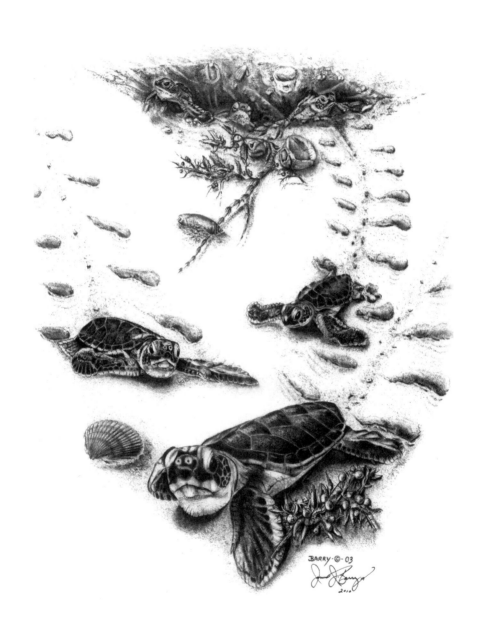

BARRY · © · 03

CHAPTER TWO

How Fish Consumption Affects Human Health

I n this book's introduction, I referred to a study that linked consumption of four kinds of fish (tuna, Chilean sea bass, swordfish, and salmon) to neurological problems, cancer, heart disorders, and autoimmune and endocrine system disorders.[1] The study, which appeared in the prestigious medical journal *Annals of Internal Medicine,* generated outrage both from within the seafood industry and from scientists who are dependent on grant funding from that industry. In addition, there was objection from some medical professionals who just couldn't stomach the idea that their favorite "health food" had been outed as a poison.

Let's put the health problems associated with eating aquatic life into perspective. In this chapter, we'll review the major threats, including food poisoning, mercury, polycyclic aromatic hydrocarbons (PAHs), polychlorinated biphenyls (PCBs), and more.

Health Threat Number One: Food Poisoning

It's never been a secret that food poisoning caused by seafood consumption occurs widely and frequently, though we usually lose sight of how often because the news stories are rarely very prominent. Some health researchers have attempted to chronicle these outbreaks. For example, a study in the July 1999 issue of the *American Journal of Preventive Medicine* showed that from 1980 to 1994, a total of 339 seafood-associated outbreaks of disease from bacteria and viruses were reported in the state of New York alone, resulting in many thousands of illnesses and some deaths. Shellfish accounted for 64 percent of these outbreaks, and finfish was responsible for 31 percent of reported incidents.[2]

In a July 2002 issue of the *International Journal of Food Microbiology,* Australian researchers reported significant food poisoning incidents involving viruses and biotoxins. The highest contamination levels were found in prawns and oysters. Risk assessments done by the Centre for Food Safety and Quality at the University of Tasmania determined that these contaminants remained at high levels even after the seafood had been cooked.[3]

Many other outbreaks have been documented throughout the world. Marine scientists at the University of South Florida estimate that there are twenty thousand cases of ciguatera poisoning every year. Indeed, ciguatera poisoning is the fish-borne illness that most commonly affects humans. The poison is contracted by eating reef fish whose flesh is contaminated with toxins produced by dinoflagellates, which are plankton that live in tropical and subtropical waters. Dinoflagellates cling to algae, seaweed, and coral. They are eaten by certain fish, which are in turn eaten by larger fish. That way the toxins move up the food chain and bioaccumulate until humans consume them.

Predator species of fish such as barracuda, snapper, and moray eel are most likely to cause ciguatera poisoning, which can't be prevented by conventional cooking. In humans, the symptoms of ciguatera poisoning include neurologic disorders and side effects that resemble chronic fatigue syndrome. Other symptoms include nausea, vomiting, and diarrhea. Some people have been known to experience muscle aches, numbness, and even hallucinations. On occasion, ciguatera poisoning has been misdiagnosed as multiple sclerosis.[4]

Symptoms of ciguatera poisoning have even developed in otherwise healthy men and women following sexual intercourse if one partner has ciguatera poisoning. In breast-fed infants of affected mothers, diarrhea and rashes can occur as the toxins migrate into breast milk. Symptoms can last for years. People usually recover, though symptoms can reappear.

Still another gremlin lurking in fish is called scombrotoxin. Scombroid food poisoning, which is caused by eating spoiled fish, ranks after ciguatera as a common type of poisoning. It is usually contracted when people eat inadequately refrigerated mackerel, tuna, mahi mahi, bonito, sardines, and anchovies.

The active toxic agent in scombroid poisoning is histamine. Symptoms associated with this type of food poisoning include skin flushing, throbbing headache, burning of the mouth, abdominal cramps, nausea, diarrhea, palpitations, anxiety, and impaired vision.[5]

In addition to ciguatera and scombroid poisoning, there is the risk of shellfish poisoning, which can have neurological effects, including paralysis. Other symptoms of shellfish poisoning include diarrhea and amnesia.

When people contract food poisoning from eating seafood, the physical effects show up quickly and usually disappear within a few hours or days. By contrast, heavy metal and chemical poisoning act much more slowly, revealing their effects over months and years; ultimately, they have even more severe and long-lasting health consequences.

Health Threat Number Two: Mercury

Physicians typically advise their patients, especially those who have had a heart attack, to eat fish for its omega-3 fatty acid content. However, in a 2010 column in *Health* magazine, medical editor and physician Roshini Raj described the unintended effects of this practice. She tells the story of a patient who came to her after surviving a heart attack. Based on another physician's advice, the patient had been eating grilled tuna and started experiencing neurological symptoms. "We tested his mercury level and it was through the roof," wrote Raj. She advised readers, "If you start to experience symptoms such as tremors, vision problems, and irritability, ask your doctor for a blood-mercury check."[6]

In the same article, Raj addressed another threat from mercury: she strongly warned pregnant and nursing women to avoid mercury-laden fish. "Mercury exposure can very seriously harm the development of a fetus or young child," she said. "Don't serve it to your little ones, who can be affected by much lower levels of the metal than adults."[7]

You won't find Raj's warning posted on shelves of canned tuna in grocery stores. Warnings against mercury poisoning have not been made a public health priority, despite the fact that mercury is a neurotoxin that affects both adults and children. Furthermore, the US Food and Drug Administration (FDA) has rarely, if ever, removed any tuna from sale in the marketplace by citing a health concern, irrespective of any mercury levels that were revealed by testing. Without information about high mercury levels coming from independent researchers and private laboratories, consumers remain ignorant about their consumption risks and are playing a game of Russian roulette with their health.

Even a casual reading of studies done throughout the world over the past decade shows that mercury concentrations in fish, particularly tuna, already constitute a real and present danger. Following are four examples of studies that were conducted in four different countries in Europe and Asia.

In 2010 researchers in Taiwan at Taipei Medical University assessed the hair mercury concentrations in women of childbearing age. They also estimated the women's average fish consumption. In more than half of the women, the amount of mercury was found to be twice the safe level set by the US Environmental Protection Agency (EPA). "The high hair mercury concentrations among women of childbearing age in Taiwan are a cause for concern due to the effect on babies' brain development," noted the study authors. They went on to make this amazing and disturbing observation: "When told that some fish contain high levels of mercury that may be harmful for unborn babies, 67.6 percent of women still indicated that they would not change their amount of fish intake."[8]

In 2004 six epidemiological researchers in Japan took umbilical cord blood samples from 63 pairs of mothers and newborns. The researchers found that the mercury concentrations in red blood cells taken from babies' blood were nearly twice as high as the concentrations in the mothers' blood. "These results confirm that methylmercury, which originated from fish consumption, transferred from maternal to fetal circulation," concluded the study authors.[9]

In 2009 a team of environmental chemists assessed mercury levels in preschool children and newborns in four locations in Spain. Nearly half had higher mercury levels than safety guidelines deem permissible, and in some children the level was more than five times the safe levels set by the EPA. Subjects who ate fish four or more times a week had mercury levels that were three times higher than those who ate fish less frequently.[10]

In 2005 scientists from the Institute of Environmental Medicine in Stockholm studied methylmercury exposure in 127 Swedish women of childbearing age who ate fish. They measured contamination in both hair and blood and found that at least 20 percent of the women had mercury levels exceeding the safe levels set by the US Environmental Protection Agency (EPA). "There seems to be no margin of safety for neurodevelopmental effects in fetus for women with high fish consumption," concluded the four scientists who coauthored the study.[11]

There is a completely separate issue relating to mercury contamination in fish that deserves your attention. Even though many health-care practitioners and government agencies recommend eating fish to obtain beneficial omega-3 fatty acids, the fact is that any protective effects obtained by the omega-3s in fish are cancelled out by their mercury content. Two studies from Finland make this case persuasively. In the first study, published in the journal *Circulation* in 1995, Finnish university health researchers examined the mercury levels and dietary intake of fish among 1,833 men (ages forty to sixty) who were free of coronary heart disease and cancer. They concluded: "These data suggest that a high intake of mercury from nonfatty freshwater fish and the consequent accumulation of mercury in the body are associated with an excess risk of acute myocardial infarction [heart attack] as well as death from coronary heart disease and cardiovascular disease."[12]

The second Finnish study was completed a decade later, with similar results. A group of 1,871 men (ages forty-two to sixty) who, like the previous group, were also free of any coronary heart disease or stroke, were tracked for nearly fourteen years. Not only was the mercury content in fish shown to be responsible for increased risk of coronary problems and death, but mercury was also found to undermine any protective effects of fish on cardiovascular health.[13]

After reading this information, you may never again be tempted to eat seafood and risk mercury's ill effects. Should you ever waver, this fact might deter you: no US federal agency regularly tests for mercury in seafood. To underscore this point, Kate Mahaffey, the late EPA research scientist who studied mercury in fish, told the *New York Times*: "We have seen exposures occurring now in the United States that have produced blood mercury a lot higher than anything we would have expected to see. And this appears to be related to consumption of larger amounts of fish that are higher in mercury than we had anticipated."[14]

If you think that tuna and other fish are less toxic when cooked, think again. The heat from cooking removes almost none of the heavy metal contaminant content in fish.

Health Threat Number Three: Polycyclic Aromatic Hydrocarbons (PAHs)

What are PAHs, and why should we be concerned? Think colon cancer. Here's how the peer-reviewed science journal *Mutation Research* describes this toxin and the way it is formed: "Polycyclic aromatic hydrocarbons, of which benzo(a)pyrene is the most commonly studied and measured, are formed by the incomplete combustion of organic matter. A number of them are carcinogenic and mutagenic, and they are widely believed to make a substantial contribution to the overall burden of cancer in humans. Cooking processes can generate PAHs in food. PAHs can also be formed during the curing and processing of raw food prior to cooking. Diet is the major source of human exposure to PAHs."[15]

Scientific studies examining the PAH content in various fish species have reached some disturbing conclusions. In 2006 Spanish researchers discovered that sixteen different types of PAHs were present in numerous species, including salmon, swordfish, mackerel, tuna, sardines, and shrimp. Of all groups tested, women and girls who ate these species had the highest PAH concentrations in their blood, meaning they had an increased risk of developing cancer.[16]

Also in 2006, Italian scientists studied the levels of PAHs in Atlantic salmon fillets and detected eleven types of these compounds in raw and smoked samples. Six of the PAH compounds existed at similar levels in both the raw and smoked fish, whereas five were sharply elevated in the smoked fish, showing that smoking creates PAHs in fish flesh. "Results confirm that PAH concentrations in smoked fish are the product of both sea pollution and the smoking process," concluded the researchers.[17]

Health Threat Number Four: Polychlorinated Biphenyls (PCBs)

PCBs are among the most environmentally persistent compounds ever created by industrial chemists. Starting in the 1920s, manufacturers began to use PCBs in many products, including transformers. Although PCBs were banned in 1976 in the United States as part of a global phaseout of the "dirty dozen" most toxic chemicals, these industrial lubricants and insulators still exist in the environment, frequently working their way up the food chain into humans. PCBs can also still be found in old electrical and industrial equipment.

PCBs are fat-soluble compounds. When they are absorbed by fish and humans, they persist in fat tissues. PCBs cause cancer, and some of these compounds can cause neurotoxicity and endocrine disruption in humans. (See chapter 4 for more about endocrine disruption.)

"Exposure to PCBs suppresses the immune system, thereby increasing the risk of acquiring several human diseases," noted David O. Carpenter in the journal *Reviews on Environmental Health*.[18] "PCB exposure, especially during fetal and early life, reduces IQ and alters behavior. The PCBs alter thyroid and reproductive function in both males and females and increase the risk of developing cardiovascular and liver disease and diabetes. Women are at high risk of giving birth to infants of low birth weight who are at high lifetime risk for several diseases."

Medical studies have found fish consumption to be a primary source of PCBs in human beings. Following are examples of the health risks associated with PCB absorption and some of the research that has been conducted.

Memory and learning impairment. Researchers assessed the blood PCB levels in 180 Michigan residents (ages forty-nine to eighty-six). The blood levels of the 101 subjects who ate fish from Lake Michigan were compared to those of 79 people who did not eat fish. Afterward, all study participants completed a battery of cognitive tests. Fish eaters had much higher levels of PCBs in their blood and much lower scores on the tests for memory and learning. "These results are consistent with previous research showing an association between in utero PCB exposure and impairments of memory during infancy and childhood," observed the seven study coauthors.[19]

Diabetes and cardiovascular disease. A study of diabetes prevalence among Native Americans in the Great Lakes region of the United States and Canada found that 20 percent of the 352 adults tested had a form of diabetes. Blood samples also showed a significant association with the levels of PCBs they had absorbed from their fish-based diet.[20]

A second study of 335 adult Mohawks found a relationship between PCBs in the blood and heart disease. "The results of this study are consistent with the conclusion that PCBs, acting through P450 enzymes, are directly responsible for increased synthesis of cholesterol and triglycerides, substances known to be major risk factors for cardiovascular disease," wrote the study's coauthors.[21]

Cancer and salmon consumption. To assess the levels of dioxins, furans, PCBs, and chlorinated pesticides in salmon, a group of scientists analyzed farmed salmon from eight regions of Europe, North America, and South America. (See chapter 6 for more about the health threats from farmed fish.) The scientists then compared the results with EPA standards for developing fish consumption advisories. According to these guidelines, individuals who ate farmed salmon from Northern Europe more than once every five months were elevating their cancer risk. People who ate salmon from North or South America more than once a month also appreciably raised their risk of contracting cancer.[22]

Health Threat Number Five: Dioxins

One hundred fifty or so individual compounds of the dioxin family form during high-temperature waste treatment and industrial processes, such as during the burning of chlorine-containing substances. Dioxins persist in the environment for decades, and even very low levels of concentration can cause harm in humans and animal life. Dioxins are known to be potent cancer agents, for example. They also can cause reproductive and developmental disorders, and they disrupt the function of the endocrine and immune systems.

Air currents widely disperse dioxin particles, which end up getting attached to the soil and to water sediments, where they are absorbed by aquatic life. Dioxin particles accumulate in fatty tissues and march up the food chain until they take up residence inside human body fat, sometimes persisting for a lifetime. Fish are particularly prone to harboring dioxin particles, largely because they circulate hundreds of gallons of water through their gills each day.

Dioxins are found in beef, pork, chicken, and almost all animal-based foods that contain fat. The greatest amounts, however, are found in farmed salmon. A study published in a 2006 edition of *Environmental Research* offered this finding: "The levels in the farmed and market salmon that we have analyzed are higher than those in almost all other foods."[23] (See chapter 6 for more about the dangers of eating farmed fish.)

Health Threats from Other Chemicals and Combinations

Fish eaters should be equally concerned about the rising tide of other chemical contaminants that are now regularly detected in aquatic life. Take flame retardants, otherwise known as polybrominated diphenyl ethers (PBDEs), for example. A 2003 Spanish study published in the *Journal of Agricultural and Food Chemistry* found fish and shellfish to be the primary human dietary sources of flame retardants. These substances disrupt the human thyroid gland and the brain, resulting in behavioral changes and hyperactivity. In children, they are associated with developmental problems and lowered IQ.[24]

Another threat comes from the mostly unknown health effects of eating fish and absorbing combinations of disparate chemicals, including PCBs. A team of scientists from the National University of Singapore's Department of Chemistry analyzed the toxins in twenty different types of seafood. They detected numerous chemicals, from flame retardants to PCBs. Three in particular stood out and were discussed in the February 2005 issue of the *Journal of Toxicology and Environmental Health*: "Daily intake of DDTs, heptachlor [an insecticide], and PCBs in seafood exceeded the conservative cancer benchmark concentrations set by the EPA, suggesting that significant numbers of people are potentially at risk."[25]

There Is Something Else Growing in Aquatic Life

A story in a May 2011 issue of *Discover* magazine gave the mainstream public its first inkling about a newly identified but growing threat to human health. The newcomer is a toxin called beta-methylamino-L-alanine (BMAA), which humans can absorb by eating fish and shellfish. BMAA is an environmental toxin produced by cyanobacteria, a common component in the diet of lake and ocean creatures. The article stated: "There's a trail of clues linking something in seafood to ALS, Alzheimer's, and Parkinson's disease."[26] ALS stands for amyotrophic lateral sclerosis, which is more commonly known as Lou Gehrig's disease.

Blooms of cyanobacteria have been occurring more frequently over the past few decades in both salt water and freshwater because of increasing temperatures (perhaps a by-product of the greenhouse effect) and contamination by sewage and agricultural chemical runoff. As fish consume the cyanobacteria, they accumulate BMAA, and that accumulation biomagnifies when larger fish consume smaller fish.

Once absorbed by humans, BMAA becomes a neurotoxin that is stored in the brain and becomes a trigger for neurological diseases, in particular, Alzheimer's disease, Parkinson's disease, and ALS. A University of Miami research team took twenty-four samples from twelve Alzheimer's patients and discovered BMAA in twenty-three of them. Other tests on thirteen ALS patients revealed that all of the subjects had the neurotoxin in their bodies.[27]

Other University of Miami researchers tested Florida's aquatic life for the neurotoxin and found the highest levels in largemouth bass, pink shrimp, and blue crabs. Lower but still significant levels were detected in oysters and mussels. The search expanded to Chesapeake Bay, where similarly high levels of the neurotoxin turned up in seafood.[28] The first overseas study of the neurotoxin was done in Sweden in 2010, when high levels were measured in fish from the Baltic Sea.

What we are seeing with this newly discovered neurotoxin, much as we have seen with PCBs and other man-made chemicals, is more evidence that human actions are warping natural ecosystems. Whether the culprits are BMAA neurotoxins, PCBs, flame retardants, or other lab-designed toxins that contaminate ecosystems and the life within them, we are seeing and feeling firsthand the results of poisoning nature's bounty.

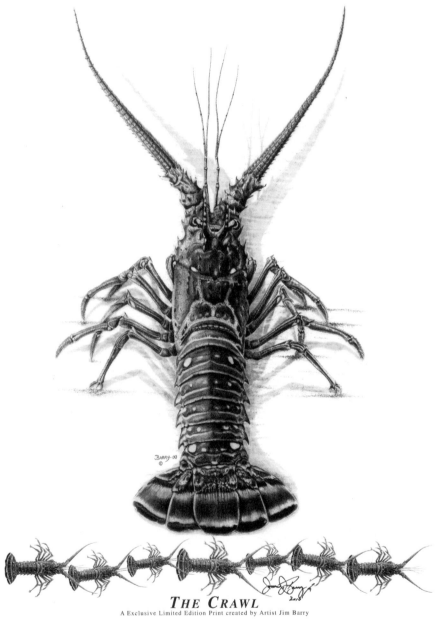

THE CRAWL
A Exclusive Limited Edition Print created by Artist Jim Barry

CHAPTER THREE

Guess What Is Really in Sushi

I f you've ever eaten in a sushi restaurant, the employees probably greeted you in unison with the traditional Japanese welcome: *irashaimase* (pronounced ee-ra-shy-ma-she). While this friendly welcome is appealing, the real draw for many sushi customers is their perception that raw and semiraw seafood, particularly fish, provides a healthful alternative to a Western diet heavily laden with red meat. This assumption can be dangerous.

Sushi consumers in the United States and other Western countries typically choose from a variety of raw fish, either served atop rice or rolled in rice and wrapped in a type of sea vegetable called nori. Rolled sushi varieties commonly include salmon (called Philadelphia, Seattle, Alaska, or BC rolls) and tuna (called Hawaiian, Jerusalem, or Western spicy tuna rolls). The omnipresent California roll contains crab or imitation crab along with avocado, cucumber, and *tobiko* (fish eggs).

Sushi is almost always served with wasabi, a sharp-tasting condiment made from a plant root, but most consumers don't realize that wasabi has a very specific role. Because of its antimicrobial properties, wasabi is served with sushi to help reduce the risk of illness from food poisoning. A 2004 study in the *International Journal of Food Microbiology* describes how all parts of the wasabi plant, including the roots, stems, and leaves, show strong bactericidal activity in laboratory experiments, primarily because of the allyl isothiocyanate levels that are present in the plant.[1] Learning wasabi's real function, as a microbe killer in sushi, should be the first red flag about the potential health risks of eating fish in the raw.

Though the Japanese have eaten sushi for many centuries, what we now find served in sushi restaurants in the United States and other countries is really a form of fast food that was first created in the nineteenth century. This relatively new variety isn't fermented like traditional sushi. The word sushi actually means "sour," reflecting its roots as a fermented form of fish packed in rice and vinegar.

Truth be told, as this chapter will graphically attempt to do, what sushi connoisseurs now eat can best be characterized as "Frankenfish." It's polluted by a toxic chemical cocktail of heavy metals, pesticides, and other industrial pollutants accompanied by vast hardy breeds of parasites and pathogenic bacteria, which thrive when they can leap up the food chain to establish a residence inside your gastrointestinal tract. Wasabi, despite its antimicrobial properties, can't compete with some of the pathogens that are now appearing in the fish pulled from our heavily polluted oceans.

Mercury, One of Sushi's Dirty Little Secrets

Evidence that shows just how toxic sushi really is has been accumulating rapidly over the past several years and should sound an alarm for every current or prospective sushi consumer. A newspaper reporter decided to take samples of tuna sushi from twenty restaurants and stores in New York City and have the fish tested for mercury by researchers at a medical laboratory. The results, which were published in the January 23, 2008, edition of the *New York Times*, revealed that one-fourth of the samples contained mercury levels so high that the US Food and Drug Administration (FDA), if it were so inclined, could have taken action under existing laws to remove the sushi from sale as a public health hazard.[2] People who eat six or more pieces of this sushi in one week seriously endanger their health, and yet the typical sushi eater consumes more than six pieces in just one meal!

Most of the tuna sushi sampled happened to be bluefin, which is generally more expensive. Because bluefin tuna is a large predator, it absorbs and accumulates additional mercury from the fish that it consumes. A person who eats just six pieces of this tuna sushi would be exposed to an alarming forty-nine or more micrograms of mercury.[3]

These findings shouldn't come as a surprise. Both the FDA and the US Environmental Protection Agency (EPA) issued a warning in 2004 that children, and women who wanted to have children, should limit their canned tuna consumption, as this form of tuna contains high mercury levels that could damage the human nervous system. Other studies have found that the amount of mercury in canned tuna could raise the risk of cardiovascular disease.

The mercury levels found in the bluefin tuna sushi in New York City were even higher than those found in canned tuna. When the tuna sushi testing results were published, one of the scientists involved, Michael Gochfeld, professor of environmental and occupational medicine at the Robert Wood Johnson Medical School, commented, "No one should eat a meal of tuna with mercury levels like those found in the restaurant samples more than about once every three weeks." Other toxicologists warned that this frequency might be too great for anyone who wanted to avoid health consequences.[4]

In an accompanying *New York Times* article, New Yorkers reacted to these revelations about hazardous mercury levels in sushi with a range of concerns, though some professed nothing more than indifference. Fifty-two-year old Paul Sohmer quipped: "At our age, I don't think it matters too much." However, this dismissive sentiment wasn't shared by younger people, such as twenty-seven-year-old Benedicte Jourdois, who took the news more seriously: "Maybe I did more damage eating sushi than eating burgers." Forty-five-year-old Bruce Seeliger added: "If it gets to the point where it's really harming people, there will obviously be lawsuits."[5]

Curious as to whether the New York City results might be replicated elsewhere, Gochfeld and four Columbia University researchers did additional mercury testing, this time with other types of tuna and in other parts of the nation. They collected one hundred tuna sushi samples from fifty-four restaurants and fifteen supermarkets in three states (New York, New Jersey, and Colorado). In addition to bluefin tuna, they also tested bigeye and yellowfin, two other tunas that commonly show up as delicacies in sushi restaurants.

The scientists summarized their findings in the October 23, 2010, issue of the journal *Biology Letters*: "Excessive ingestion of mercury—a health hazard associated with consuming predatory fishes—damages neurological, sensory-motor, and cardiovascular functioning. The mercury levels found in bigeye tuna (*Thunnus obesus*) and bluefin tuna species (*Thunnus maccoyii*, *Thunnus orientalis*, and *Thunnus thynnus*) exceed or approach levels permissible by Canada, the European Union, Japan, the United States, and the World Health Organization."[6]

Their paper goes on to say, "The mean mercury concentrations of all samples exceed the concentration permitted by Japan and the maximum daily consumption considered safe by the US Environmental Protection Agency. Mean mercury levels for bluefin akami exceed those permitted by the US Food and Drug Administration, Health Canada, and the European Commission. On average, one order of bigeye tuna sushi, the species used most often for sushi, exceeds the safe maximum daily dose recommended by Health Canada and the safe limit established by the WHO [World Health Organization] and FAO [Food and Agricultural Organization] for women of childbearing age."[7] As for yellowfin tuna sushi, the researchers reported total mercury levels that were significantly higher than those found in samples obtained by the FDA in 2004.

What are the health implications for people who consume tuna sushi with this level of mercury? According to these scientists, the health risks based on medical study results from the past decade include neurodevelopmental defects such as mental retardation, cerebral palsy, deafness, blindness, dysarthria, and adult neurocardiovascular toxicity.

There is also the risk of cancer to consider. Environmental health researchers at the State University of New York at Albany issued the following warning to a physician who wrote about sushi for the British newspaper the *Daily Mail* in April 2006: "If you eat a meal of salmon sushi more than twice a year, you will increase your risk of cancer. The contaminants found in fish often overpower its supposed beneficial effects. People think they're improving their health by eating sushi, but they are in fact poisoning themselves."[8]

PCBs, Dioxins, and Other Chemicals Lurk Here Too

In addition to mercury, increasingly heavy loads of industrial chemicals, including PCBs, dioxins, flame retardants (PBDEs), and pesticides, are found in both ocean-caught tuna and ocean-caught and farm-raised salmon, which are used to make sushi. "Once eaten," warns British physician and health columnist Danny Penman, "these poisons stay in the body for decades, reducing fertility and steadily weakening the immune system and potentially causing cancer."[9]

Over the past decade, research teams at various US universities have conducted more than a dozen major studies that measured and compared the contaminants that bioaccumulate in ocean-caught and farm-raised fish, including many species commonly used for sushi. One group of researchers published their conclusion in a 2010 issue of the journal *Reviews on Environmental Health*: "The problem is that most fish have at least some degree of chemical contamination with methylmercury (which binds to muscle), and/or with persistent organic pollutants such as dioxins, polychlorinated biphenyls, polybrominated diphenyl ethers, and cholorinated pesticides (which concentrate in fish fat). These chemicals have adverse effects on nervous system function, modulate the immune system, and are associated with elevations in the risk of cardiovascular disease."[10]

Some sushi proponents claim that PCB and PBDE levels are lower in wild salmon than in farmed salmon, and the contaminants can be reduced still further in both raw and cooked fish by removing the skin. Researchers at the Marine Environmental Research Institute in Maine have dispelled both of these misleading notions. The researchers published their findings in the April 2008 issue of the journal *Chemosphere*: "Total PBDE concentrations in the farmed salmon were not significantly different from those in the wild Alaskan chinook samples." They also reported that removing the fish's skin resulted in no overall reduction in the contamination levels, and, in some cases, PBDE concentrations were higher in samples with the skin off.[11]

A Whole Family of Bacteria Moves In

In 2008 researchers from the Institute for Food Quality and Food Safety in Hanover, Germany, tested 250 sushi samples that were taken from sushi bars and fish retailers.[12] The researchers identified the following bacteria in some of the samples: *Escherichia coli*, salmonella, *Staphylococcus aureus*, and *Listeria monocytogenes*. Once ingested, any of these microbial pathogens are capable of wreaking havoc on the human gastrointestinal tract.

You have probably heard about the threats posed by E. coli and salmonella, both of which can cause humans much gastrointestinal misery, if not death, but what about the other two pathogens that were found—*Staphylococcus aureus* and *Listeria monocytogenes*? The first is the most common cause of staph infections in humans, and the second causes listeriosis, which kills up to 30 percent of people who are infected by it. Some of the bacteria detected in the German study may have come from cross-contamination that occurred when the sushi was prepared.

During the first decade of the twenty-first century, periodic outbreaks of microbial food poisoning from sushi consumption were reported worldwide. For example, during March and April 2004 in Queensland, Australia, thirteen people (ages twenty to thirty-nine) came down with salmonella poisoning as a result of eating sushi rolls.[13] No one died, but all the victims suffered for at least five days from severe stomach cramping, diarrhea, and vomiting.

Several years earlier, a microbiological survey of sushi done by the Australian Capital Territory government found that 31 percent of sushi samples were contaminated with potential food-borne pathogens at levels outside of acceptable microbiological limits for ready-to-eat foods.[14] This finding should have been a warning of the poisoning that was to come.

Parasites Seek a Mortgage on Your Intestinal Home

Tiny but potentially deadly worms in sushi enter the human intestinal tract in one of two ways: as live worms hiding in fresh sushi, or as dead worms in sushi fish that has been frozen. Even when dead, these worms can trigger symptoms in humans that include severe stomach pain that persists for days.

Parasites love laying eggs in fish flesh and excel at remaining hidden and undetected while colonizing their human prey. We humans provide ideal hosts because our bodies offer a steady supply of nutrients. In addition to gastrointestinal problems, the presence of parasites can affect the human mind, both emotionally and cognitively, and worsen asthma and allergies.

Anisakid nematodes are worms that usually are hidden in the flesh of salmon, sardines, squid, and cuttlefish. These parasites infect the human gastrointestinal tract when ingested, and residues left by the worms in fish flesh can trigger allergic reactions in humans. Health problems caused by these parasites include violent abdominal pain, nausea, vomiting, muscle weakness, numbness, increased heart rate, irritability, and symptoms that mimic Crohn's disease. In addition, all parasite infestations weaken the immune system.

The first case of poisoning from anisakid nematodes was documented fairly recently, in the 1960s in Holland. Since then, untold numbers of cases have been recorded on all five continents as the popularity of sushi has spread. A 2010 study in the *International Journal of Food Microbiology* reported that anisakis type I larvae were found in 74.3 percent of tested fish from the seas of Japan.[15]

Diphyllobothrium is a fish tapeworm that can live for up to twenty years inside the human intestinal tract and can grow to several dozen feet in length. It's mostly found in salmon from North America and parts of Europe and Asia, though it sometimes also shows up in trout and perch. Besides sushi, other dishes that feature uncooked fish, such as *ceviche* from Latin America and *tartare maison* from France, can play host to this parasite.

Symptoms of diphyllobothriasis in humans include the usual poisoning symptoms, such as abdominal pain, diarrhea, fatigue, vomiting, weight loss, and compromised immunity. In addition, the parasite's presence in the small intestine can produce anemia because it can absorb 80 percent or more of the B_{12} vitamins in the human body.

Now, after you have read this chapter, do the parasites and other contaminants identified in sushi spoil your appetite for it? Does the potential negative effect on your health diminish your enthusiasm for this raw dining fare? Do you still retain your taste and desire for sushi? If the answer is yes, then you are indeed a glutton for punishment!

How To Do a Parasite (or Bacteria) Cleanse

Even a cursory Internet search will turn up dozens of parasite cleanse techniques and products that could be helpful in ridding your body of creepy critters that you have unknowingly given an intestinal home. Sometimes, parasites can be detected during a colonic cleanse done by a qualified colonic therapist. Usually, however, a parasite's presence becomes obvious only when the physical symptoms become severe and can be readily diagnosed. A microscopic analysis done by a skilled practitioner can confirm an amoeba or parasite infestation.

Herbs that are commonly used in parasite-cleansing programs include clover seed and wormwood. Hippocrates Health Institute uses a product called LifeGive Par-A-Gon, which is made exclusively for the institute.

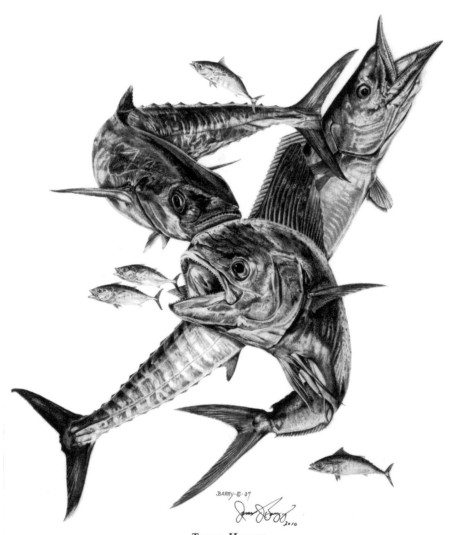

BARRY·©·07

2010

TRIPLE-HEADER

CHAPTER FOUR

Sexual Disruption in Fish Threatens Humans

When the first public warning about a looming health threat was issued by a group of wildlife biologists in 1991, few people in the media or the government took notice. During a weeklong work session on endocrine-disrupting chemicals, this group of expert scientists concluded the following: "Many compounds introduced into the environment by human activity are capable of disrupting the endocrine system of animals, including fish, wildlife, and humans. Endocrine disruption can be profound because of the crucial role hormones play in controlling development."[1]

Since this early alarm was sounded, scientific findings about endocrine-disrupting chemicals and their effects on reproductive health have become impossible to ignore. The impact is being seen and felt worldwide. Like the proverbial canaries in a coal mine, fish and other aquatic life are the first casualties in this massive human experiment with nature.

The culprits are a class of chemicals known as endocrine disrupters, which commonly appear in consumer products, prescription drugs, and pesticides and are the by-products of industry. They act like estrogens, which is to say, they mimic the effects of natural estrogens in the body. They frequently make their way into the world's water supplies, where they are absorbed by aquatic life and begin their travels up the food chain to humans. Endocrine disruptors first affect males, regardless of species, because they are more sensitive to estrogenic influences.

"Some of the first eerie signs of a potential health catastrophe came as bizarre deformities in water animals, often in their sexual organs," observed Nicholas D. Kristof, a columnist for the *New York Times*, in a June 27, 2009, column. He wrote: "In the Potomac [River] watershed near Washington, male smallmouth bass have rapidly transformed into 'intersex fish' that display female characteristics. This was discovered only in 2003, but the latest survey found that more than 80 percent of the male smallmouth bass in the Potomac are producing eggs. Now scientists are connecting the dots with evidence of increasing abnormalities among humans, particularly large increases in numbers of genital deformities among newborn boys."[2]

Pharmaceutical Drugs in Fish Multiply

As scientific testing for the presence of synthetic chemicals in water has become more sophisticated during the twenty-first century, entirely new categories of chemicals are being detected in aquatic life. In particular, the newfound residents include pharmaceuticals that are widely prescribed to treat depression, psychiatric disorders, high blood pressure, allergies, cholesterol, and a range of other human ailments. A study published in the December 2009 edition of the journal *Environmental Toxicology and Chemistry* revealed that fish caught around wastewater treatment plants in five large US cities (Dallas, Phoenix, Philadelphia, Chicago, and Orlando) all contained combinations of at least seven pharmaceutical drugs and several chemicals from personal care products.[3]

Wastewater treatment plants are unable to eliminate these chemicals, which are excreted in human waste. Fish that live downstream from wastewater treatment plants are constantly exposed to contaminated water, and as a result they are rendered unfit to eat, though state and local government agencies usually don't bother to issue permanent health advisories warning fishermen and fish consumers.

Canadian researchers who studied the St. Lawrence River near Montreal detected significant quantities of antidepressants in fish, and the drugs seem to be affecting the fish in numerous ways. "We have data that does show that antidepressant drugs do accumulate in fish tissues—there's significantly more in the liver than in the muscle, but there's [even] more in the brain tissues," reported Sébastien Sauvé, the chemist who coauthored the study, which appeared in the April 2011 issue of the peer-reviewed journal *Chemosphere*.[4]

Though he didn't see an immediate threat to people who eat these fish, Sauvé did note that one in four people living in Montreal are known to be consumers of antidepressant or antipsychotic drugs. The result is that the body burden caused by these chemicals being absorbed by fish continues to intensify, which, according to Sauvé, has an impact on the river's ecosystem, and perhaps other unpredictable consequences that we can only begin to speculate about. (Body burden is a term that means a buildup of heavy metals and synthetic chemicals in human or animal bodies.)

It's no stretch of the imagination to say that these drugs will bioaccumulate in the tissue of people who absorb them from drinking the water and eating the fish. And as discussed in chapter 2, the bioaccumulation of dozens of chemicals from multiple sources leads to numerous human health repercussions.

Drugs in US Waterways Lead to Widespread Fish Horrors

US Geological Survey studies show that most bodies of water in the United States are now contaminated with pharmaceuticals. Why? Because wastewater treatment plants cannot remove the drugs before releasing "purified" water back into the environment.

The cost of implementing reverse osmosis and other sophisticated processes to remove synthetic chemicals would be astronomical and could bankrupt most local governments.

More than one hundred new drugs enter the marketplace each year. The health effects of these drugs, combined with the thousands of chemicals already in the environment, remain mostly unknown. Because many human diseases have long latency periods, it is difficult to connect an illness or disorder with exposures from long ago. Also complicating the matter is the fact that some of the drugs in our waterways act upon more than one hormonal pathway in the human body and are absorbed through multiple exposures from water, food, and air.

In September 2006, the *Washington Post* featured a front-page article revealing the findings of the US Geological Survey, which tested rivers in the Washington, DC, area. The rivers provide the tap water for several million residents of DC, northern Virginia, and suburban Maryland. Here are the key findings:[5]

- At least 80 percent of the bass caught in these rivers and river tributaries and then tested were found to have intersex organs, with the males growing eggs in their reproductive organs.
- Since 2003, when these abnormalities in fish were first discovered in the upper Potomac River and West Virginia, the incidence of intersex births has spread rapidly and widely.
- Hormone-disrupting chemicals released by wastewater treatment plants into these rivers were identified as the probable culprits behind these abnormalities.
- The problem may be "a result of several pollutants acting in combination," according to scientists. In other words, chemical synergies may be producing these mutant strains of fish.

In 1996 the US Congress directed the US Environmental Protection Agency (EPA) to develop a screening program to identify which chemicals were causing fish abnormalities. Today, more than a decade later, the EPA hasn't tested a single chemical. The agency claims this costly technological challenge is beyond its limited resources. Scientists interviewed by the *Washington Post* expressed shock at the spread of hormone-disrupting chemicals and the EPA's inability to even study the problem, much less offer solutions. Equally shocking is the confession by a water utility spokesman, who admitted ignorance as to whether or not water purification plants could remove the mutation-causing chemicals before humans ingested the water, or even if the utility is analyzing the water to look for the right things.[6]

A 2007 US Geological Survey analysis of rivers surrounding Portland, Oregon, long known as one of the "cleanest" cities in the United States, revealed a dramatic accumulation of designer synthetic chemicals in the mud of the Willamette and Tualatin Rivers and several creek tributaries. Drugs detected at high levels read like someone's science experiment with a home medicine cabinet: there were three antidepressants, a mood stabilizer, an antibiotic, an antifungal used to treat athlete's foot, high blood pressure medications, sedatives, antibacterial agents found in detergents, a fungicide . . . the list goes on and on.

"So little is known about what they [the chemicals] do to fish and aquatic life that no one is sure what's safe in the environment over the long term," reported the *Portland Oregonian* newspaper in a March 2008 article. "Scientists were surprised by what they found. Scientists working on related studies found signs that something in the water is turning the bodies of local salmon haywire. Young male and female salmon from the Willamette River around Portland held traces of an egg yolk protein usually found only in adult female fish beginning to develop eggs."[7]

Endocrine-disrupting chemicals were found in all but one of the twenty-three river sites where the scientists took samples. The newspaper reported: "Combined with PCBs, flame retardants, and other pollutants already known to be present in local rivers, the drugs and other substances put fish at risk in various ways, such as possibly disrupting their immune systems." None of the experts interviewed could even begin to speculate on the possible health risks of eating the contaminated fish or drinking the contaminated water.[8]

A Worldwide Overview of Reproductive Harm

The United States is not the only country where waterways are polluted with endocrine-disrupting chemicals. Contamination has been reported by scientists all over the world. Following is a sampling of research results.

China. Beijing University scientists studying the Japanese medaka fish species shared these findings in 2008: "DDE, the major and most persistent metabolite of DDT, was continually detected in wild fishes that showed abnormal gonad development, such as intersex." The scientists also found that when DDE coexists with other endocrine-disrupting chemicals, the resulting synergies accelerate and intensify endocrine disruption.[9]

Europe (continent-wide). Dutch public health researchers reviewed studies done in Europe throughout the 1990s and found a clear pattern of endocrine-disrupting chemicals adversely affecting a variety of fish species. They reported: "The observed abnormalities vary from subtle changes to permanent alterations, including disturbed sex differentiation with feminized or masculinized sex organs, changed sexual behavior, and altered immune function."[10]

Ireland. In the Shannon International River Basin District, which encompasses eleven rivers, the effects of endocrine-disrupting chemicals on feral brown trout were investigated in 2010. Among the estrogenic chemicals identified in the water were phthalates and an alkylphenol. (Phthalates are used as solvents in such products as perfumes and cosmetics, while alkylphenols, a family of surfactants, appear in detergents and other products.) This study not only confirmed the presence of estrogens in the rivers but also found that 100 percent of the male brown trout sampled at some sites showed either endocrine disruption or intersexuality.[11]

Italy. A team of nine biologists from the University of Genoa reviewed recent studies that showed that bisphenol A (BPA) together with other estrogenic chemicals may be responsible for the disrupting effects observed in fish in the Po River. BPA is a plasticizer used in cosmetics, personal care products, and baby bottles. It is also used to line food cans. After exposing common carp for two weeks to BPA concentrations known to exist in the river, the scientists reported: "In carp males, BPA caused severe alterations of testis structure . . . a few carp also showed intersexuality (27 percent) and . . . a significant reduction of testosterone was observed in both males and females."[12]

North Sea. Endocrine disruption was detected in North Sea cod and flatfish at even higher levels than had previously been measured in English Channel and Irish Sea fish. This was considered highly unusual because these North Sea fish don't have proximity to land or known sources of endocrine disrupters. Such a finding strongly suggests that a gradual accumulation of these chemicals occurs as a result of larger fish feeding on smaller fish that contain the chemicals.[13]

South Africa. Along three sites of the Luvuvhu River in Limpopo Province, samples of an indigenous fish species (*Oreochromis mossambicus*) were collected and analyzed. Between 48 percent and 63 percent of the fish from those sites were intersex individuals.[14] In addition, the insecticide DDT and its metabolites DDE and DDD were detected in fat samples from fish at all three testing sites.

Even Tiny Amounts Cause Problems

Scientists in Canada intentionally added synthetic estrogen to a remote lake and set in motion a chain reaction of mutations in the native fish population. According to results reported in a May 2007 issue of the journal *Proceedings of the National Academy of Sciences*, the experiment demonstrated that even low levels of estrogen in municipal wastewater can cause wild fish populations to mutate and collapse.[15]

Biologists with the Canadian Rivers Institute at the University of New Brunswick injected synthetic estrogen (the type found in birth control pills) into a Canadian lake to test the hypothesis that endocrine-disrupting chemicals secreted from human bodies can disrupt fish populations. After the first summer of exposure to these chemicals, male minnows in the lake began producing egg proteins. Then their sperm cells became undeveloped, and the males began producing eggs as well. This impaired ability to reproduce resulted in a collapse of the lake's minnow population in the second year of the study. As *National Geographic News* reported, "The population even failed to recover in the two years after the researchers stopped adding estrogen, indicating the effects were quite persistent."[16]

"Low concentrations of an estrogen can have very dramatic, very severe effects on fish reproduction," remarked Karen Kidd, a biologist and the study leader. She believes that if her team had continued adding the endocrine disrupter to the lake, it would have had a similar impact on larger and longer-lived fish, such as trout.

It's important to note how this feminization of males is occurring among aquatic species other than fish. Clams, for instance, are especially sensitive and vulnerable to endocrine-disrupting chemicals, even at tiny exposure levels. A September 2006 study in the journal *Biological Letters* revealed that intersex characteristics in clams (*Scrobicularia plana*) were appearing within the same

United Kingdom marine ecosystems where "extensive feminization of male fish in UK rivers has been shown to occur."[17] A 2009 issue of *Ecotoxicology and Environmental Safety* presented a study from Portugal, which showed that up to 71 percent of clams collected from the Guadiana River had intersex development, which coincided with the detection of several endocrine-disrupting chemicals in the water.[18]

As the 2006 book *The Hundred Year Lie* points out, humans excrete dozens of different types of endocrine-disrupting synthetic chemicals, just as potent as birth control pills, into the planet's bodies of water each and every day. These amounts are constantly increasing, and the mutations we see among aquatic life appear to be indicators of subtle changes already happening within humans.[19]

Chemicals in Sunscreens Cause Reproductive Disorders

Have you ever applied a sunscreen to your skin and then minutes later jumped into a lake or the ocean? If you have, it's time to consider the unintended consequences your actions are having on aquatic life.

That sunscreen you used likely contained a chemical called oxybenzone, which helps you to tan but is also a documented hormone disrupter, similar to estrogen in its effects on humans and other life forms. Even when you simply take a shower after using a sunscreen, you wash oxybenzone down the drain, where it travels unscathed through wastewater treatment plants and into the nearest bodies of water.

Studies conducted by the US Centers for Disease Control and Prevention in 2005 found oxybenzone in the bodies of 97 percent of 2,500 US residents whose blood had been tested at random. Once in lakes, rivers, or oceans, oxybenzone settles into sediments and gets absorbed by small fish as they feed. The small fish are eaten by larger fish, a process that biomagnifies the oxybenzone up the food chain. Another common chemical found in sunscreens, octyl-methoxycinnamate, also acts as a hormone disrupter; both chemicals have been detected in human breast milk, likely as a result of biomagnification.

As the prominent toxicologist Samuel Epstein points out in his book *Toxic Beauty*, a pregnant woman's absorption of these two chemicals can "release these feminizing ingredients through the placenta into unborn children, increasing the prospect that male babies will be feminized or will develop hormone imbalances later in their lives."[20]

In 2005, two separate studies done in California and Switzerland discovered oxybenzone in various fish species and sediments. Researchers from the University of California, Riverside, examined fish and sediments collected near wastewater outfalls serving the city of San Diego and the counties of Orange and Los Angeles. They found oxybenzone, along with alkylphenols (endocrine disruptors) and 17beta-estradiol (a form of estrogen), in all samples. This finding corresponded with the observation that two-thirds of the males in two coastal fish species had become feminized and carried ovary tissue.[21]

Marine biologists in Switzerland tested fish from a river and several lakes for the presence of oxybenzone and three other UV filter compounds used widely in sunscreens, cosmetics, shampoos, and hair sprays. All four compounds were detected. The study authors concluded that recreational activities, such as using sunscreens while sunbathing, played a major role in the release of these chemicals, as did discharges from wastewater treatment plants.[22]

Summary of Hormon-Altering Chemicals

Eight hormone-altering chemicals or groups of chemicals are now commonly found in fish and other aquatic life. These are toxins to be concerned about if you consume fish or drink tap water.

1. Alkylphenols. A family of organic compounds, alkylphenols are used as precursors to detergents, as additives for lubricants and fuels, in fragrances for consumer products, and in fire-retardant materials. They have been used by industry for at least four decades. Lawmakers in the European Union enacted restrictions on the sale and use of certain alkylphenols due to their toxicity, persistence, and ability to bioaccumulate. No similar warning or action has been taken by regulatory agencies in the United States.

Scientists have recently developed tests that are sensitive enough to identify and measure the presence of alkylphenols in aquatic life. In one study, white suckerfish were collected upstream and downstream of the wastewater treatment outfall in Boulder, Colorado. The scientists who conducted the study had this to say about their findings: "Gonadal intersex, altered sex ratios, reduced gonad size, disrupted ovarian and testicular histopathology, and vitellogenin induction consistent with exposure to estrogenic wastewater contaminants were identified in white suckers downstream from the wastewater treatment outfall and not at the upstream site. Chemical analyses determined that the effluent contains 17beta-estradiol, alkylphenols, and bisphenol A. These results indicate that the reproductive potential of native fishes may be compromised."[23]

2. Bisphenol A. Also known as BPA, bisphenol A is a chemical compound used to make polycarbonate plastic. On January 15, 2010, a report by the US Food and Drug Administration raised concerns that BPA can harm children and fetuses. Subsequently, Canada's government listed BPA as a toxic substance. Studies have shown that BPA affects the growth and reproductive capacity of aquatic life. In a study published in a 2010 edition of *Environmental Toxicology and Chemistry*, BPA was found in two Canadian rivers. It was also found that 85 percent of the fish population was female.[24]

Denmark was the site of one of the first comprehensive studies of BPA in fish. The researchers reported: "Females with male germ cells among the normally developing oocytes were observed in all groups, in up to 50 percent of the female fish, independently of exposure regimen."[25]

3. Contraceptive EE2. A synthetic estrogen, EE2 is a key component in contraceptive pills. After being absorbed by the body, EE2 is excreted through female urine and feces and passes through wastewater treatment plants mostly unaltered. Once the estrogen enters waterways, it can cause hormone disruption and intersex fish. This problem is particularly acute in countries where the use of contraceptives is widespread. By some estimates, one-third of British women between the ages of sixteen and forty-seven use the oral contraceptive pill. This is one reason why many of the scientific studies examining the effects of synthetic estrogen on aquatic life have come from the United Kingdom.

For instance, consider these research results: "In UK rivers, feminization responses, including intersex, are widespread in wild roach (*Rutilus rutilus*) fish populations and severely affected fish have reduced reproductive success. In the wild, exposure to environmentally relevant concentrations of the contraceptive estrogen 17alpha-ethinylestradiol (EE2) during early life has significantly wider implications for the sexual physiology in fish than has thus far been determined."[26]

Another study, this one from 2006, measured EE2 and other estrogens at forty-five sites on thirty-nine rivers throughout the United Kingdom. The researchers concluded: "The results provide further and substantive evidence to support the hypothesis that steroidal estrogens play a major role in causing intersex in wild freshwater fish in rivers in the United Kingdom and clearly show that the location and severity of these endocrine-disrupting effects can be predicted."[27]

4. Diazepam. A generic prescription medication, diazepam is marketed under the brand name Valium and is used to treat anxiety and insomnia. Scientists from the Mississippi State Chemical Laboratory examined catfish livers for five target compounds, including diazepam and oxybenzone. They reported, "Diazepam was detected in all ten fish liver samples."[28]

5. Polychlorinated biphenyls (PCBs). There are many types of PCBs, and about 130 of these chemical substances have been used in fluids for transformers and capacitors, especially electrical transformers, as plasticizers in cements and paints, and as coatings on electrical wiring. PCBs are found everywhere in the industrialized world, and many are highly toxic substances that cause neurotoxicity and endocrine disruption when absorbed by animals and humans. Though they were first identified in 1966 by a Swedish chemist as an environmental danger, it wasn't until 1979 that the US Congress banned the domestic production of PCBs. It has since been discovered that PCBs persist in the worldwide environment for decades, particularly in marine sediments and the fatty tissues of living organisms.

Here is a description of just one of many studies that demonstrate the endocrine disruption caused by PCBs: "Largemouth bass and common carp were collected from thirteen sites located in the Mobile, Apalachicola-Flint-Chattahoochee, Savannah, and Pee Dee River Basins to document spatial trends in accumulative chemical contaminants, health indicators, and reproductive biomarkers. Mercury and polychlorinated biphenyls (PCBs) were the primary contaminants of concern. Concentrations of mercury in bass samples from all basins exceeded toxicity thresholds for piscivorous mammals, juvenile and adult fish, and piscivorous birds. Total PCB concentrations may be a risk to piscivorous wildlife. Intersex gonads were identified in 42 percent of male bass representing twelve sites and may indicate exposure to potential endocrine-disrupting compounds."[29] (Piscivorous is a term used to describe animals that feed on fish.)

6. Pesticides and insecticides. Among organochlorine compounds that kill insects by disrupting their nerve cells, the best known may be DDT. A Swiss chemist was awarded the Nobel Prize in 1948 for discovering DDT, which was introduced as an allegedly safer alternative to the arsenic and lead compounds previously used to control insects on croplands. Once it was understood that DDT and related compounds—including aldrin, dieldrin, mirex, and toxaphene—bioaccumulate in the fatty tissues of living organisms and then biomagnify up the food chain to cause reproductive harm, legislative steps were taken to restrict their production and use.

There are far too many studies to list here that document the bioaccumulation of these persistent chemicals in fish. To illustrate the extent of the problem, let's consider a major 2007 study from the US Geological Survey. Carp, black bass, and channel catfish were collected from fourteen sites along the Colorado River Basin. Concentrations of formerly used organochlorine pesticides, such as toxaphene and dieldrin, were detected in the fish. Researchers noted that intersex fish were found at seven of fourteen sites and included smallmouth bass, largemouth bass, catfish, and carp, indicating exposure to these endocrine-disrupting compounds. They stated: "A high proportion of smallmouth bass from the Yampa River (70 percent) were intersex."[30]

7. Selective serotonin reuptake inhibitors (SSRIs). A class of antidepressants called SSRIs is prescribed to treat anxiety, depression, personality disorders, and severe insomnia, though the drugs have also been prescribed off-label to treat irritable bowel syndrome. SSRIs increase the extracellular level of serotonin and are marketed worldwide under such brand names as Lexapro, Prozac, Paxil, and Zoloft. Their effectiveness was called into question by a huge study presented in the January 2010 *Journal of the American Medical Association.* The study concluded: "The magnitude of benefit of antidepressant medication compared with placebo may be minimal or nonexistent, on average, in patients with mild or moderate symptoms."[31]

Not until 2005 did scientists investigate the increased levels of SSRI chemicals in fish. In that year a team of scientists from

Baylor University took samples of four fish species from a stream in north Texas and found the generic SSRIs fluoxetine and sertraline and the SSRI metabolites norfluoxetine and desmethylsertraline.[32] Two years later researchers in Canada took fish samples from Hamilton Harbour in Lake Ontario and detected the generic SSRIs fluoxetine and paroxetine, and the SSRI metabolite norfluoxetine.[33]

8. Triclosan. First put into commercial use in 1972, triclosan is an antifungal and antibacterial agent used in dozens of consumer products, such as mouthwash, shaving cream, toothpaste, and deodorant. Once released into the environment, triclosan reacts to sunlight to form other, more toxic compounds, including dioxins. A highly persistent compound, it has been detected in marine sediments that are more than three decades old. Numerous studies indicate that triclosan is an endocrine disrupter that chemically mimics the thyroid hormone. It also has proved toxic to aquatic bacteria and the algae responsible for much of the planet's photosynthetic activity.

Only in the past couple of years have scientists begun to study the presence of triclosan and related chemicals in marine environments. It's clear from the studies conducted thus far that triclosan isn't removed from wastewater by wastewater treatment plants. Baylor University chemists in 2009, for instance, sampled rivers and fish near treatment facilities in Chicago, Dallas, Orlando, Phoenix, and West Chester, Pennsylvania. Trace levels of triclosan were found everywhere in the rivers and sampled fish, along with many other personal care product chemicals and pharmaceuticals.[34]

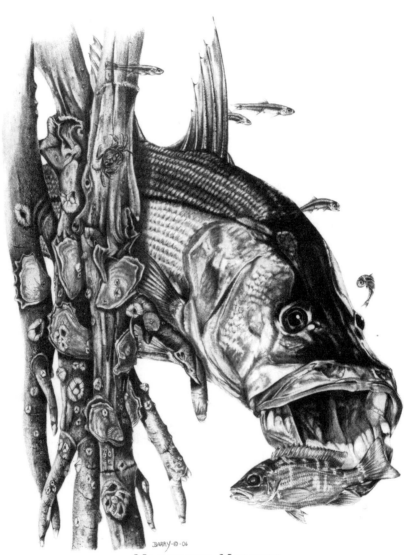

BARRY · © · 06

MANGROVE MOMENT
A Exclusive Limited Edition Print created by Artist Jim Barry

CHAPTER FIVE

The Omega-3 Health Argument Is Fishy

We've all heard it. Eat more fish! Eat more fish! Get your daily minimum requirement of essential omega-3 fatty acids by eating more fish! They're rich in omega-3s! But what are the facts behind all of this rhetoric?

The American Heart Association urges all adults to eat oily fish at least twice weekly to reduce their cardiovascular disease risk. Other public health organizations and government health agencies make similar recommendations. But what health risks are they overlooking, and why are they overselling the benefits of consuming fish?

You won't hear any debate from me about the importance of omega-3 fatty acids for human health. Our bodies cannot produce omega-3s, so we must get them from food sources. But over the past half-century, omega-3s have been crowded out of our diet by the less healthful omega-6 fatty acids that are found in meat, cooking oils, and processed foods.

There are three kinds of omega-3 fatty acids. The first two, eicosapentaenoic acid (EPA) and docosahexaenoic acid (DHA), can both be synthesized in the human body from the third kind, alpha-linolenic acid (ALA). This is an important point to emphasize, and I will come back to it later: ALA can be obtained from plants, and it's all you need. ALA provides the human body with the other two types of omega-3s. You don't need fish or fish oils.

The health benefits of consuming omega-3 fatty acids are well documented. According to research scientists at the Linus Pauling Institute at Oregon State University, many medical studies have concluded that omega-3 fatty acid intake helps reduce the risk of cardiovascular disease. Omega-3 intake also has been found to decrease the risk of heart attack and other sudden heart conditions. In addition, Alzheimer's disease and dementia might be triggered in people who don't consume enough omega-3s.

Beyond preventing some health problems, omega-3 fatty acids can also alleviate existing problems. For example, increasing fatty acid consumption helps treat type 2 diabetes and lower elevated serum triglycerides. In addition, studies indicate that omega-3 fatty acids may be beneficial in treating depression, bipolar disorders, and even schizophrenia. Omega-3s also decrease joint tenderness in rheumatoid arthritis patients, and they are considered important for visual and neurological development in infants, who can get these fatty acids from mother's milk.

Mainstream medical practitioners usually recommend that we consume 300 to 400 milligrams of omega-3 fatty acids every day to absorb the amounts we need to bolster immune system health and prevent the range of diseases triggered by omega-3 deficiencies. But where should we get the omega-3s that we need? Are fish the only and best source? Or has the public been sold on consuming a product based on vested economic interests, rather than real, scientific data?

Most consumers aren't aware that the omega-3 fatty acids found in fish aren't produced by fish. These fatty acids are produced only by plants. When small fish eat marine algae, they absorb the algae's omega-3 fatty acids, and when large fish gobble up the small fish, they absorb the fatty acids stored in the smaller fish. This process continues up the food chain, until humans consume larger, cold-water fish, such as herring, salmon, and albacore tuna, which contain high concentrations of bioaccumulated fatty acids.

There is evidence that consuming fatty acids from fish raises the risk of contracting coronary heart disease, rather than lowers it, as is commonly proclaimed in so much health-related information today. The earliest research emerged in a 1997 study done in Finland, which examined 21,930 men (ages fifty to sixty-nine) who had no history of cardiovascular disease. It so happened that these men were smokers, so it's conceivable there was an interaction between eating fish and smoking cigarettes, but since the study authors focused on the omega-3 fatty acids in fish, we have evidence for an association with heart disease that can't be overlooked. Here is what the research team found: "The intake of omega-3 fatty acids from fish was directly related to the risk of coronary death. . . . The hypothesis that frequent intake of fish is protective of coronary heart disease has recently been challenged by three recent prospective studies."[1]

Plant sources of omega-3 fatty acids carry no associated health risks. Of all the plants and nuts containing omega-3s, the richest source of this essential nutrient is marine algae. Studies of human subjects who took marine algae supplements determined that they are a safe, convenient, plant-based source of DHA. In addition, there is evidence that these supplements are easily absorbed by the human body, and they may be absorbed even more efficiently when taken with meals.[2]

So my strong advice to you is to cut out the middleman (fish) and go right to the source (marine algae) for your omega-3 needs. Eating fish for their omega-3 content is a little like using an intermediary every time you want to withdraw money from your own bank account. Using an intermediary is inefficient. The same holds true when you keep fish in your diet. Consuming fish or fish oil taxes your well-being and adds nothing to your health that you can't get from more healthful and risk-free sources.

Some Fish Harbor Dangerous Fatty Acid Combinations

A cheap fish is becoming a staple in the diets of low-income people. It's called tilapia, and consumption in the United States alone doubled between 2003 and 2010. Possible reasons are that tilapia is easy to produce in large quantities on fish farms, and it thrives by consuming inexpensive corn-based feeds. Yet this newly popular farmed fish poses a bigger risk of heart disease than even pork or hamburger. Why? Because tilapia contains very low levels of beneficial omega-3 fatty acids but very high levels of omega-6 fatty acids. This imbalance, contributes to heart disease and other health problems.

This problem is not exclusive to tilapia but also extends to farmed catfish, as was discovered by a team of researchers from the Wake Forest University School of Medicine. The results were published in a 2008 edition of the *Journal of the American Dietetic Association.*[3] The researchers examined tilapia and catfish from seafood distributors that supply supermarkets and restaurants. The fish came from fish farms in several nations and from two South American enterprises that operate international fish distribution companies. All of the samples had been frozen in preparation for gas chromatography analysis of their fatty acid levels.

Here is what one of the researchers told *Science Daily*: "The recommendation by the medical community for people to eat more fish has resulted in consumption of increasing quantities of fish such as tilapia that may do more harm than good."[4] In both farmed tilapia and catfish, the ratio of omega-6s to omega-3s is 11:1, compared to a 1:1 ratio in salmon. Omega-6 fatty acids contribute to the narrowing of coronary arteries, which is a major risk factor for heart attacks in humans.

Floyd Chilton, a senior author of the study and a professor of physiology and pharmacology at Wake Forest, criticized health organizations for advising consumers to eat more fish. He said,

"The classical Hippocratic admonition is 'First, do no harm.' I think it behooves us to consider this critical directive when making dietary prescriptions for the sake of health. Cardiologists are telling their patients to go home and eat fish, and if the patients are poor, they're eating tilapia. And that could translate into a dangerous situation."[5]

What About Fish Oil Supplementation?

By now, you know that consuming fish presents a risk to your health because of all the harmful elements they possess, including chemical pollutants and unwanted fats, that can be passed on to you. Still, some people believe it's okay to use fish oil supplements instead of eating fish to get higher levels of omega-3 fatty acids in their diet. There are many reasons why this is not a safe bet.

Whenever oil is extracted from fish and exposed to air for any length of time, it becomes rancid. Fish oil oxidizes as soon as it's exposed to oxygen, light, or heat. To extract oil from fish, the entire fish is usually minced, and the oil is extracted using heat and chemical solvents. This process can sometimes create carcinogens, which are left as by-products in the oil.

Fish oil processors usually disguise the dead fish smell by adding antioxidants and preservatives. Some processors also try to remove the chemical contaminants, such as mercury and dioxins, in the fish, which diminishes omega-3 content. They then seal the fish oil in gel capsules so the smell can't escape. Break open one of these capsules sometime. The rancid odor will assault your sense of smell. (Be warned that fish oil occasionally shows up as an additive in margarine and shortenings produced by major food companies.)

A healthful alternative to fish oil has always been flaxseed oil, which became a fixture in the pantheon of health elixirs as far back as 650 BC when Hippocrates lauded its many therapeutic uses. You don't have to use flaxseed oil to get the health benefits of flax.

Alternatively, you can eat the flaxseeds themselves—either raw, sprouted, or ground up and sprinkled on salads—to get the highest possible concentrations of omega-3s. Chia seeds and hempseeds can be used in the same way.

Fish Oil Linked to Increased Colon Cancer Risk

Fish oil is often promoted by mainstream doctors as a good source of omega-3 fatty acids for people who are at risk of inflammatory bowel diseases. The problem is, fish oil increases the risk of colon cancer and severe colitis. Evidence of this link emerged late in 2010, and many medical practitioners, not to mention consumers, are still unaware of the connection.

Nutrition scientists at Michigan State University hypothesized that feeding fish oil enriched with DHA to mice would decrease their cancer risk. This was a common assumption among mainstream nutrition researchers. What the scientists found, however, was the exact opposite of what the researchers believed to be true. "Our findings support a growing body of literature implicating harmful effects of high doses of fish oil consumption in relation to certain diseases," commented Jenifer Fenton, the food and human nutrition scientist who led the research team.[6]

Science Daily reported these findings with stark language: "The research team found an increase in the severity of the cancer and an aggressive progression of the cancer in not only the mice receiving the highest doses but those receiving lower doses as well."[7] It took only four weeks for the tumors to develop in the mice as a result of the increased inflammation caused by the fish oil. While it's certainly true that these alarming findings were the result of an experiment using lab animals, the mouse has proven over time to be a good indicator of potential disease effects in humans.

This research underscores the dangers of using high doses of fish oil, despite the recommendation of the fish oil manufacturing industry. By some estimates, the recommended doses are twenty times or more what the average person needs. These high levels may be producing overdose reactions in the human body.

A decade before these findings about cancer were released, British researchers with the Institute of Human Nutrition discussed the negative effects of fish oil supplementation and how it could raise the risk of cancer in humans at the International Society for the Study of Fatty Acids and Lipids conference in Japan. It's remarkable to me that so much time elapsed before additional research showing a possible cancer link was undertaken, given what's at stake for human health.

Clearly we need to pay close attention to these cancer findings. This is especially true if you use, or have ever used, high levels of fish oil in the belief that its omega-3 content would be beneficial to your health.

Fish Oil Harms Athletic Performance

It may be a challenge for many people to connect the dots between optimal physical exercise and their consumption of fish oil, but that's just what a team of French medical researchers did in 2003. Their findings, which were published in the *British Journal of Nutrition*, should be of concern to any aspiring athlete: fish oil supplementation reduces exercise effectiveness.

The researchers came to this conclusion by measuring exercise performance in a group of men. For the twenty days before the test, each man took six grams of fish oil per day. The researchers found that fish oil supplements decrease fuel production in the muscles during exercise. This decrease in energy could negatively affect the performance of any competitive athlete, whether a cyclist, runner, or bodybuilder.[8]

Six Common Fish Oil Myths Debunked

1. Fish oil benefits pregnant women. Producers and purveyors of fish oil products have promoted the idea that their supplements can help pregnant women avoid postpartum depression, while simultaneously promoting the cognitive development of their unborn children. Medical researchers in Australia proved this claim to be false in a 2010 study that tested the response of 2,400 pregnant women to fish oil. The women were randomly assigned to take either 800 milligrams of DHA from fish oil per day or placebo capsules containing vegetable oil. Six months after the women gave birth, the rates of postpartum depression were no different between the two groups, indicating that fish oil had no beneficial effect. In addition, the children of women from the two groups did not score any differently at age eighteen months on a battery of tests designed to show whether the mother's intake of fish oil had been beneficial to them while still in the womb. The fish oil industry ignored these findings.[9]

2. Fish oil slows mental decline. Another marketing claim trumpeted by the fish oil industry is that fish oil slows the onset of mental decline associated with Alzheimer's disease. Still another 2010 study has demolished this contention. Funded by the National Institute on Aging and published in the *Journal of the American Medical Association*, the study randomly assigned four hundred men and women in their mid-seventies who were likely to have Alzheimer's to either a placebo group or a group that took two grams of DHA from fish oil per day. After eighteen months, there was no difference in the degree of mental decline between the two groups, as measured by a rating scale and mental testing.[10]

Here is the specific language the study authors used to describe their conclusion about the DHA in fish oil: "Supplementation with DHA compared with placebo did not slow the rate of cognitive and functional decline in patients with mild to moderate Alzheimer's disease. . . . The hypothesis that DHA slows the progression of mild to moderate Alzheimer's disease was not supported, so there is no basis for recommending DHA supplementation for patients with Alzheimer's disease."[11] That clearly tells us that fish oil should not be touted as a preventative for cognitive deterioration and age-related decline.

3. Fish oil strengthens the immune system. Many mainstream physicians love to believe this one, though they seem vague on the details of how it is supposed to happen. We all know how important our immune systems are: they play an indispensible role in preventing illness and disease. So why would you knowingly and consciously engage in an activity that weakens your immune system and makes life-threatening health problems more likely? Supplementing with fish oil may be doing exactly that.

There are a number of ways that omega-3 derivative fish oils weaken our immune systems according to research presented by the International Society for the Study of Fatty Acids and Lipids during a 2000 conference in Japan. These initial findings were documented and expanded in a 2003 study published in the prestigious journal *Lipids:* "High fish oil intake may not be beneficial long term; i.e., it may compromise host immunity and may address only the secondary consequences of immune activation in some clinical conditions."[12]

4. Fish oil can prevent cancer. This myth is founded on a huge reservoir of wishful thinking, stirred up by the fish oil manufacturing industry. Several studies in major peer-reviewed medical journals have disproved the theory that fish oil prevents cancer. Let's focus on one of them, published in a 2006 edition of the *British Medical Journal.* Thirteen British researchers reviewed nearly one hundred studies that had been conducted worldwide on omega-3 fatty acids and cancer prevention. From this wealth of research, an inescapable conclusion emerged: "We found no evidence that omega-3 fats had an effect on the incidence of cancer, and there was no inconsistency."[13]

5. Fish oil prevents artery inflammation. You've probably heard this one, too, and wouldn't it be wonderful if it were the truth? Imagine clearing your arteries of inflammation-causing plaque every time you took a fish oil supplement. In a 2004 study published in *Current Atherosclerosis Reports,* several researchers reviewed the available evidence and reported this finding: "Fish oil did absolutely nothing significant to decrease the inflammation as evidenced by the failure of CRP [C-reactive protein] to decrease. . . . There was no evidence for an anti-inflammatory effect as judged by CRP levels."[14]

6. Fish oil supplementation can prevent heart disease. The widely held view that taking fish oil can decrease your risk of cardiovascular disease persists despite numerous well-designed studies that contradict this notion. In 2010 researchers at the University of Pittsburgh Graduate School of Public Health presented findings to the American Diabetes Association that showed that consuming more omega-3 fatty acids from fish doesn't lower heart disease risk in women with type 1 diabetes. People with this type of diabetes are generally at much greater risk of developing heart disease, so this population was ideal for determining whether fish oil can stop or reverse the buildup of plaque in the arteries.[15]

These findings supported previous research, such as the 2002 study in the journal *Cardiovascular Research* that examined the effect of omega-3s from fish on cerebral arteries and the incidence of stroke. According to the authors, both the fish oil groups and the control groups showed close to equal atherosclerotic progression: "In this group of selected patients with documented coronary artery disease, omega-3 PUFA [polyunsaturated fatty acids] given for two years did not demonstrate an effect on slowing progression of atherosclerosis in carotid arteries as measured by ultrasound."[16]

An earlier study from 1999 that was published in the *Annals of Internal Medicine* examined whether omega-3s from fish or fish oil capsules could prevent atherosclerosis. After two years, researchers concluded that arterial clogging had worsened in both the fish oil group and the placebo control group. Of the forty-eight patients in the placebo group, forty-one showed disease progression based on coronary angiography measurements. Among the fifty-five patients in the fish oil group, thirty-nine showed disease progression.[17]

A US study involving a great number of subjects examined whether increasing fish in the diet decreased the risk of coronary heart disease. Researchers tracked 44,895 male health professionals (ages forty to seventy-five) over a six-year period using validated dietary questionnaires. Here is what the Harvard School of Public Health research team concluded in 1995: "These data suggest that increasing fish intake from one to two servings per week to five to six servings per week does not substantially reduce the risk of coronary heart disease among men who are initially free of cardiovascular disease."[18]

Finally, in case you need even more evidence, here is another fish oil study to think about. University of Wales College of Medicine researchers studied 3,114 men (age seventy and younger) who complained about angina. They were divided into four groups: group one was advised to eat two portions of oily fish each week or to take three fish oil capsules daily; group two was advised to eat more fruit, vegetables, and oats; group three was asked to do what both groups one and two were doing; and group four was given no specific dietary advice.

At years three and nine of the study, mortality among the four groups was determined. The researchers found that the risk of cardiac death was higher among subjects who had been advised to eat oily fish, and the risk for sudden cardiac death was even greater. Furthermore, this excess risk was largely seen among the subgroup given fish oil capsules. These results, which were published in the *European Journal of Clinical Nutrition*, led the British researchers to this disturbing and inescapable conclusion: "Men advised to eat oily fish, and particularly those supplied with fish oil capsules, had a higher risk of cardiac death."[19]

Plant-Based Sources: Solving the Omega-3 Puzzle

Why fish oil can't possibly work as claimed was the subject of an intriguing article in the science journal *Explore*. The article was researched and written by Brian Peskin, a former professor in the Department of Pharmacy and Health Sciences at Texas Southern University. Peskin made a strong case that fish oil supplements supply EPA and DHA in greater amounts than the human body can ever naturally produce—or effectively absorb—on its own.[20] This overdosing would help to explain why fish oil might worsen the condition of diabetic patients by raising their blood sugar levels and thwarting the insulin response. It also explains why fish oil causes other health problems.

The article makes a strong case that using fish oil supplements is a misguided attempt to correct essential fatty acid deficiencies in mainstream diets, which are based on processed foods. Because Peskin found that the constituents of fish oils "are far from being correct physiologically for most (human) tissue," he created a plant-based formula that is more functional and better absorbed by the human body.[21] The article also describes the importance of a substance Peskin calls parent essential oils (PEOs), which are the building blocks of all the omega-3 fatty acids. Peskin defines PEOs as unadulterated oils that contain fatty acids but have not been subjected to chemical processing or excessive heat treatments.

In the June 2011 edition of his newsletter, *Second Opinion*, physician Robert Rowen wrote about PEOs and analyzed Peskin's argument. Rowen described a study that used a medical device called a digital pulse analyzer to measure the effects of plant-based PEOs on the human arterial aging process. The research sample included thirty-five people (thirteen males and twenty-two females, age seventy-five and younger) who took PEOs. Half took the PEOs for less than twenty-four months, and half took them for a longer period. In twenty-five of the test subjects, arterial flexibility, a key determinant of heart disease risk, improved. Overall, the subjects' mean biologic arterial age dropped by nearly nine years, which is truly remarkable.[22]

Here's how Rowen characterized the results: "PEOs are so called because they are the eighteen carbon chain fatty acids that are the only true 'essential fatty acids.' The longer-chain fatty acids of marine oils, including EPA and DHA, are not 'essential' fatty acids. Your body makes these longer-chain fatty acids automatically from the true parent essential oils—if you're getting enough of the PEOs. We've come to believe that somehow humans don't automatically make sufficient longer-chain fatty acids [EPA and DHA] from the parent oils. We do!!! And this study proves that it's better to let your body make what it needs in its own wisdom, than to force-feed it what it might not want or need."[23]

"The tragedy," continued Rowen, "is that fish oil taken in the amounts that most physicians recommend can overdose you with 20 times too much DHA and 250 to 500 times too much EPA. Just think what would happen if you took 250 aspirin capsules—you'd be dead. Of course, fatty acids are not a drug like aspirin. But anything can act like a drug in your body if you take it in pharmacological amounts. That's my concern about the unbridled rise of marine oil consumption. We just don't know what [it] will do in the long run."[24]

This research underscores that fish oil doesn't provide the eighteen carbon-chain fatty acids known as parent essential oils. In fact, there is evidence that fish, krill, and oils from other marine animals contribute to the oxidation process that is a major cause of vascular disease.

Table 3. Plant-based sources of omega-3 fatty acids (ALA)

Food	Serving	Alpha-linolenic acid content (in grams)
Flaxseed oil	1 tablespoon	7.3
Walnuts, English	1 ounce	2.6
Flaxseeds, ground	1 tablespoon	1.6
Walnut oil	1 tablespoon	1.4
Soybean oil	1 tablespoon	0.9
Mustard oil	1 tablespoon	0.8
Walnuts, black	1 ounce	0.6

Source: Linus Pauling Institute, Oregon State University

Instead of Fish Oil: Chia Seeds

When people ask me about a healthful replacement for fish and krill oil, I suggest they try a proprietary blend of chia seeds produced by a company called Mila. I've recommended this product for several years, and I've seen resounding health benefits from this balanced omega-3 and omega-6 food. Check it out in the supplements store at hippocratesinst.org.

More on Plant-Based Sources

It's ironic, even strange, that mainstream nutritionists note that marine algae produces the omega-3s that fish bioaccumulate, yet they fail to acknowledge that marine algae can be the most direct and natural food source of these essential fatty acids. It's as if these traditionalists are so fixated on the alleged health advantages of fish that they have never imagined that green and blue algae could be a human food source. Maybe these so-called experts are so stubborn in their own dietary habits that their professional judgment has become impaired.

Nutritionists also overlook several other foods that are sources of omega-3 fatty acids: chia seeds, raspberry seeds, walnuts, Brazil nuts, sesame seeds, avocados, and dark leafy green vegetables, such as kale, spinach, and collard greens. One of the best ways to get ample amounts of omega-3s in your diet is to eat combinations of these foods in large quantities as often as possible. Let's take a closer look at three of the top plant-based omega-3 sources: marine algae, spinach, and walnuts.

The Health Benefits of Marine Algae

No longer considered just "pond scum," blue-green algae, also known as cyanobacteria, has achieved new respectability as a healing agent and a source of healthful nutrients, including omega-3 fatty acids. These algae can be found in both seawater and freshwater environments.

Spirulina, when sold in digestible forms, is a therapeutic type of blue-green algae. Two species—*Arthrospira platensis* and *Arthrospira maxima*—are now being used as dietary supplements. Spirulina is rich in protein (up to 77 percent by dry weight) and contains all the essential amino acids, making it a complete protein. It also has thiamine, riboflavin, nicotinamide, pyridoxine, folic acid, and vitamins C, D, A, and E.

Chlorella is a single-celled green algae that contains the photosynthetic pigments chlorophyll a and b. It also is a complete protein. Dried chlorella is composed of nearly 50 percent protein and 10 percent vitamins and minerals. The remaining content is fats and carbohydrates. Chlorella acts as a detoxifier when absorbed by humans. In addition, chlorella's ability to reduce cholesterol and high blood pressure and to enhance the immune system has been proved in scientific experiments.

In a three-volume series that I authored, *Food IS Medicine: The Scientific Evidence,* I collected thousands of peer-reviewed medical studies showing the healing powers of various plant foods, and marine algae turned out to be the most powerful healing agent of all. About forty-five different medical conditions, from cancer to diabetes, can be prevented or treated using marine algae. Here are some examples of the research I found in scientific journals:

• *Nutrition,* 2009. Key finding: "Chlorella supplementation resulted in the conservation of plasma antioxidant nutrient status and improvement in erythrocyte [red blood cell] antioxidant enzyme activities in subjects. Therefore, our results are supportive of an antioxidant role for chlorella and indicate that chlorella is an important whole-food supplement that should be included as a key component of a healthy diet."[25]

• *Journal of Medicinal Food,* 2009. Key finding: "In humans, *Spirulina maxima* intake decreases blood pressure and plasma lipid concentrations, especially triacylglycerols and low-density lipoprotein cholesterol, and indirectly modifies the total cholesterol and high-density lipoprotein cholesterol values."[26]

• *Journal of Medicinal Food,* 2001. Key finding: "These findings suggest the beneficial effect of spirulina supplementation in controlling blood glucose levels and in improving the lipid profile of subjects with type 2 diabetes mellitus."[27]

• *Annals of Nutrition and Metabolism,* 2008. Key finding: "The results demonstrate that spirulina has favorable effects on lipid profiles, immune variables, and antioxidant capacity in healthy, elderly male and female subjects and is suitable as a functional food."[28]

• *IBC Library Series,* 1998. Key finding: A team of medical researchers at Royal Victoria Hospital in Canada examined how Super Blue-Green Algae strengthens the human immune system.

In this double-blind study, fifty people consumed 1.5 grams of this algae. As a result, their natural killer cell activity increased significantly, provoking these immune cells to move from the bloodstream into body tissues to scavenge for sick cells and toxic invaders.[29]

The Health Benefits of Spinach

Spinach, one of the most nutritious of all vegetables, contains high levels of antioxidants and vitamins A, C, E, and K, along with zinc, iron, selenium, folic acid, and numerous other nutrients in addition to omega-3 fatty acids. Medical studies have documented that spinach consumption reduces the risk for at least nine types of cancer. Here are three representative studies that show the health benefits of eating spinach:

• *Journal of Neuroscience,* 1998. Key finding: Spinach may be beneficial in retarding functional age-related cognitive behavioral deficits and may have some benefit in combating neurodegenerative disease.[30]

• *Asia Pacific Journal of Clinical Nutrition,* 2008. Key finding: Spinach was one of the top candidates among twenty-two dietary sources tested for the potential to treat secondary complications of diabetes.[31]

• *Oncology Reports,* 2005. Key finding: Spinach may suppress tumor growth by suppressing angiogenesis and might be one of the best anticancer agents.[32] (Angiogenesis refers to the formation of blood vessels.)

The Health Benefits of Walnuts

English walnuts are known to contain higher concentrations of omega-3 fatty acids than any other type of nuts. In addition, walnuts boast high levels of protein, magnesium, phosphorous, potassium, and such vitamins as A, B_{12}, C, D, and E. Here are some noteworthy research findings about walnuts:

• *European Journal of Clinical Nutrition,* 2009. Key finding: Walnuts produced significant reductions in fasting insulin levels, an effect seen largely in the first three months of use.[33]

• *American Journal of Cardiology,* 2006. Key finding: Sources of plant-derived omega-3 fatty acids include walnuts. Because of the remarkable cardioprotective effects of omega-3 fatty acids, consumption of food sources that provide them should be increased in the diet.[34]

• *European Journal of Clinical Nutrition,* 1998. Key finding: Walnuts in the diet showed changes that might be expected to reduce the risk of cardiovascular disease.[35]

• *Nutrition and Cancer,* 2008. Key finding: Research mice that were engineered to develop cancer were fed a diet including walnuts (amounts equivalent to two ounces a day for humans) and were compared to mice that were fed a similar diet without walnuts. The mice that ate walnuts were less likely to develop breast tumors. After 145 days, 100 percent of the mice that were not fed walnuts had developed cancer, whereas only 50 percent of the mice that ate walnuts had developed cancer.[36]

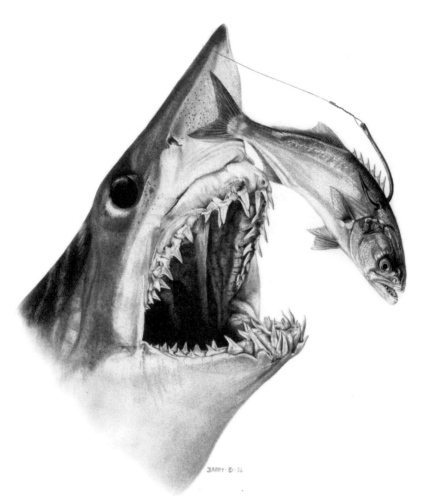

BLUE WATER BITE
A Exclusive Limited Edition Print created by Artist Jim Barry

CHAPTER SIX

The Big Myth: Farmed Fish Are Safer Than Wild

A lot of people believe that eating farm-raised fish is a more healthful choice than consuming wild-caught fish, especially those lifted from our sewer-dump oceans. The reasoning goes like this: because aquaculture (also known as aqua farming) involves raising fish under controlled conditions, in which both the environment and feed quality are regulated, there is less chance that farmed fish will be contaminated with the same alarming range of toxins as wild fish. This belief constitutes one of the biggest prevailing myths about aquatic life and human health.

It's virtually impossible to find untainted salmon in today's market economy. The majority of salmon sold in the United States is from commercial fish farms in northern Europe, Chile, and Canada. In most cases, consumers' efforts to identify farmed versus wild salmon are in vain. When the word "fresh" appears on the label of a salmon package, the contents are usually farm-raised rather than wild. Similarly, when the word "Atlantic" is used, the contents are almost always farmed, despite the implication that the fish came from the ocean.

Farmed Salmon and Human Health Dangers

No one has done more research to debunk the myth that farm-raised fish is a healthful choice than David O. Carpenter, a Harvard Medical School graduate who directs the Institute for Health and the Environment at the State University of New York at Albany. He and his research team have raised an urgent alarm about the safety of aqua farming. Over the past decade, they have conducted a dozen major studies and published their findings in prominent peer-reviewed medical journals. Their research has documented the increasing amounts of toxins, including dieldrin, dioxins, PCBs, and toxaphene, in farm-raised fish and their serious effects on human health.

Carpenter and his team conducted the first comprehensive global study on the health risks of eating farm-raised salmon. The study results were published in a January 2004 issue of the journal *Science* and included this conclusion: "Having analyzed over two metric tons of farmed and wild salmon from around the world for organochlorine contaminants, we show that concentrations of these contaminants are significantly higher in farmed salmon than in wild."[1] The researchers also issued this warning to consumers: "This study suggests that consumption of farmed salmon may result in exposure to a variety of persistent bioaccumulative contaminants with the potential for an elevation in attendant health risks."[2]

What should make this study even more alarming for consumers is that the tested samples, which had high levels of PCBs, dioxins, dieldrin, and other industrial toxins, came from distributors that provide salmon to eight regions around the world, including sixteen large cities in North America and Europe. Supermarkets in Paris, London, Oslo, Frankfurt, and Edinburgh sold fish containing contamination levels so high that no consumer could safely eat more than eight ounces in a month without suffering severe health consequences. The toxicity levels should have triggered a health advisory based on US Environmental Protection Agency (EPA) standards. In North America, salmon sold in Boston, San Francisco, and Toronto contained contaminant levels that exceeded safety recommendations.

"If anything, the study conservatively estimates the health risks from the contaminants in farmed salmon," said Carpenter. "The EPA fish consumption guidelines don't take into account exposures people have to the same cancer-causing substances from all other sources in the environment. They assume that fish consumption is the only source of exposure people have to these substances, and we know that's not true."[3] Carpenter noted that there is yet another drawback to using EPA safety guidelines: "The recommendations only consider the risk of cancer and don't take into account the neurological, immune, and endocrine system effects that have been associated with these contaminants."[4]

The contaminants in farmed salmon originate in the fish meal and fish oil that the salmon are fed while they are penned up. The fish meal is made of ground-up sea animals, such as krill and larger species of forage fish. A shocking fact that many consumers and even health authorities don't realize is that the same fish meal that is fed to farmed salmon is also fed to chickens and pigs. In a 2000 report on aquaculture in the journal *Nature,* the authors stated: "The poultry and swine industries are the world's largest consumers of fish meal."[5] Because toxin-laden fish meal is routinely fed to chickens and pigs, consumers of these meat products are subject to the associated health risks.

US citizens who expect the Food and Drug Administration (FDA) to protect them from the hazardous toxins in fish and other meats will find themselves sorely disappointed. "FDA regulatory levels were never designed to consider exclusively human health risks," observes Barbara Knuth of Cornell University. "The health and diet information and the technology FDA used to help set the regulatory levels for PCBs are twenty years out of date. We can detect PCBs at much lower levels today. New studies provide more information about the health risks associated with these substances, and people eat more fish today. FDA levels are inappropriate for setting fish consumption advisories, which is why these fish are still allowed to be sold legally in the United States."[6]

Fish Farm Facts

• Aquaculture has rapidly become such a profitable industry over the past three decades—averaging an 8 percent growth in the number of farmed fish every year over that period—that it now threatens to displace all traditional forms of fishing in the wild.[7]

• The fish species that are now predominantly raised on fish farms include salmon, bigeye tuna, carp, tilapia, catfish, and cod.[8]

• By 2009, more than half of all fish consumed globally was raised on fish farms.[9]

• According to a report by the National Oceanic and Atmospheric Administration, the United States imports 86 percent of its seafood from other countries, and half of that volume comes from fish farms.[10]

• China produces more than 70 percent of all fish raised in world aquacultures.[11]

• About 90 percent of all shrimp consumed in the United States is farm raised and imported.[12]

• Salmon, which is aquafarmed in great numbers, also is being genetically modified for even faster growth and higher profits.[13]

More Research Focuses on Farmed Salmon and Health Risks

In earlier chapters, the topic of heavy metal contamination, especially from mercury, in wild-caught fish is frequently discussed. Mercury contamination is a concern in farmed fish as well. A team of nine medical researchers from the University of Texas Medical

Branch examined the aquaculture industry and released their findings in the July 2009 issue of the *International Journal of Hygiene and Environmental Health*: "Although mercury contamination levels are no higher in farmed fish than in wild fish, their interactive toxic effects with coexisting man-made contaminants are not known. . . . From various estimates, consumption of these farmed fish can raise risks to health consequences, such as cancer. Such health risks may overshadow the cardiovascular benefits from the consumption of certain farmed fish [such as salmon]."[14]

Other metals are also found in the tissues of farmed fish. A study published in a 2004 edition of *Environmental Toxicology and Chemistry* revealed that concentrations of nine metals were found in farmed Atlantic salmon (*Salmo salar*) and two species of wild-caught salmon (chum and coho). Of the nine metals, organic arsenic was significantly higher in farmed than in wild salmon, whereas cobalt, copper, and cadmium were significantly higher in wild salmon.[15]

When it comes to other types of industrial toxins, there is increasing evidence that farmed fish may contain greater amounts than wild fish. Researchers analyzed samples of farmed Atlantic salmon from Maine and eastern Canada, organically farmed Norwegian salmon, and wild Alaskan chinook salmon for the presence of PCBs, dioxin-like PCBs, polychlorinated dibenzodioxins and dibenzofurans, and chlorinated pesticides. The researchers concluded: "Total PCB concentrations in the farmed salmon were significantly higher than those in the wild Alaskan chinook samples. Organically farmed Norwegian salmon had the highest concentrations of PCBs; their TEQ [toxic equivalent] values are in the higher range of those reported in farmed salmon from around the world. Skin removal does not protect the consumer from health risks associated with consumption of farmed salmon."[16]

The University of Texas Medical Branch researchers who commented about mercury content in farmed fish also commented about other toxins: "Farmed fish, although presumably safer from contamination than wild fish, have, in fact, higher body burden of certain toxic chemicals that may present health concerns to unsuspecting consumers."[17] Examples of man-made contaminants found at high levels in farmed fish include PBDEs, PCBs, pesticides, brominated flame retardants, dioxins, and antibiotics.

"Human cancer risks associated with consumption of farmed salmon contaminated with PCBs, toxaphene, and dieldrin are higher than cancer risks associated with consumption of similar quantities of wild salmon," concluded a study published in the May 2005 issue of *Environmental Health Perspectives*.[18] The study also included this finding: "Many farmed Atlantic salmon contain dioxin concentrations that, when consumed at modest rates, pose elevated cancer and other health risks. However, dioxin and dioxin-like PCBs are just one suite of many organic and inorganic contaminants and contaminant classes in the tissues of farmed salmon and the cumulative health risk of exposure to these compounds via consumption of farmed salmon is likely even higher."[19] Finally, the study ended with this disturbing cautionary note to consumers: "Although both farmed and wild salmon are sold commercially within and outside the United States, the FDA has not established a tolerance or other administrative level of dioxin-like PCBs for commercially sold fish or for other foods."[20]

In 2006, another group of researchers published a study in the journal *Environmental Research*. By applying EPA methods for developing fish consumption advisories for cancer, this team of scientists determined that contaminants in farmed salmon warranted strong warnings: To avoid an elevated risk of cancer, consumers should consume no more than one meal that includes farmed salmon from northern Europe every five months. Because farmed salmon from Chile is less contaminated, the scientists advised eating no more than one or two meals per month. They did not limit their warnings to farmed salmon: "Upon consideration of all of these organochlorine compounds as a mixture, even wild Pacific salmon triggered advisories of between one and less than five meals per month."[21]

In this study, the fish that had high levels of one of the fourteen major contaminants, such as the pesticides mirex or DDT, also were more likely to contain high levels of the other toxins. Combinations of two or more chemicals create an additional health dilemma for consumers and public health authorities. Here's what the study's authors had to say about this: "Since thirteen of the fourteen contaminants that we have reported are either known or probable human carcinogens, and since all of them have a variety of noncancerous actions, clearly if one hopes to protect against risks of cancer, noncancer effects, or both, one must deal with the fact that fish contain a chemical mixture of contaminants. Unfortunately, we have few well-developed and validated tools for evaluating health risks of chemical mixtures and inadequate information on the degree and nature of interactions among the various contaminants."[22]

When a person who eats fish is exposed to two or more of these toxins, the effects could be additive (each toxin adds to the health impacts of the other) or even synergistic (two or more toxins interact to produce effects much greater than any one can create on its own). Research evidence has found that synergies do occur between chlordane and endrin, between toxaphene and chlordane, between HCB and dioxin, and between DDE and PCBs, all of which are found in most samples of farmed salmon. Because of these powerful synergies and their potentially catastrophic effects on human health, people who consume salmon, whether farmed or wild, are taking risks with their long-term health.

Table 4. Common toxins in farmed salmon (measured in salmon samples with levels above FDA safety guidelines)

Toxin	Type	Effect
aldrin/dieldrin	pesticide	probable cancer-causing agent
dioxins	industrial chemical	probable cancer-causing agent
mirex	pesticide	probable endocrine disrupter
PBDEs	flame retardant	probable cancer-causing agent and endocrine disrupter
PCBs	industrial chemical	probable endocrine disrupter
toxaphene	pesticide	probable cancer-causing agent

Sources: [23, 24, 25]

Cramped Fish Farms Breed Viruses

Overcrowding is typical in fish-farm pens, and with it comes the rapid proliferation and spread of viruses. One of the worst outbreaks in commercial aquaculture started in 2007 when infectious salmon anemia, a viral disease, invaded all of the major fish farms in southern Chile. At last report, the virus continues to spread and wreak havoc, causing salmon production to be cut by half. Chile and Norway have overlapping aquaculture industries, partly as a result of cross-ownership, so it was no surprise when biologists traced the origin of the salmon virus to salmon eggs that were shipped to Chile from Norway, which has the largest aquaculture industry in the world.

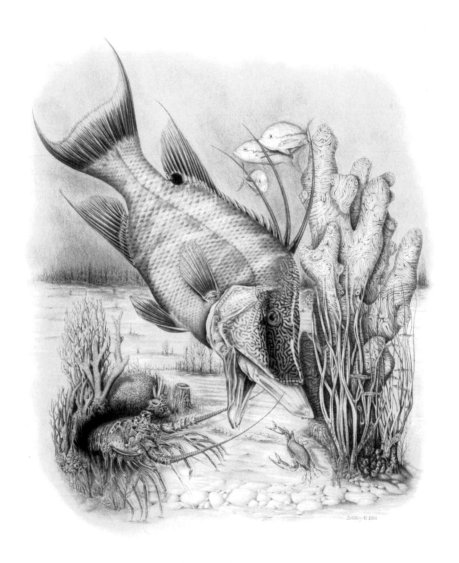

HOGFISH DELIGHT

CHAPTER SEVEN

The Overfishing
Problem, Unsolved

According to estimates made by marine biologists associated with the World Wildlife Fund and other environmental groups, the population of large oceangoing fish has declined by up to 80 percent or more over the past hundred years. This decline is the result of overfishing by the world's four million fishing vessels.[1]

Several years ago a *National Geographic* magazine article titled "Still Waters, The Global Fish Crisis" shed light on some disturbing facts. Here is a sampling: Twelve species of Mediterranean fish that were once traditionally caught for food are now commercially extinct. The population of cod, which used to be a common catch from the North Sea to New England, is in collapse. And so many fishing boats ply the waters of the Java Sea and the Gulf of Thailand that even those once abundant and seemingly endless stocks of fish are close to exhaustion.[2]

Among all of the alarms sounded about declining populations, one particularly urgent cry appeared in a November 2006 issue of the journal *Science*. The article was coauthored by fourteen marine biologists and fisheries experts from the United States, Canada, and Sweden. They wrote the following: "Human-dominated marine ecosystems are experiencing accelerating loss of populations and species, with largely unknown consequences. . . . We conclude that marine biodiversity loss is increasingly impairing the ocean's capacity to provide food, maintain water quality, and recover from perturbations."[3]

Why are we humans desecrating the ocean and decimating the life that depends on it? The never-ending slaughter of fish is driven by the fishing industry's desire for more profits and growth. It is also a by-product of misguided medical advice that encourages people to increase the amount of fish in their diets. (See chapter 2 to learn more about how eating fish affects human health.)

To help alleviate the growing shortage of wild fish, people in the fish business are relying on two innovations—fish farms and genetically modified fish that grow larger and faster. Ironically, neither development has helped wild fish or stanched their population loss. Rather, fish farming and genetic manipulation both come with significant downsides.

Aquaculture Creates More Problems Than Solutions

Tens of thousands of aquaculture farms now exist worldwide. These fish farms raise more than 220 species of finfish (most commonly carp and salmon) and shellfish (most commonly clams and mussels).[4] Aquaculture now supplies half of the total fish and shellfish for human consumption.[5] However, this statistic does not mean that wild fish are off the hook.

"Aquaculture is a contributing factor to the collapse of fisheries stocks worldwide," determined the ten coauthors of a study that was published in a June 2000 edition of the journal *Nature*. "For some types of aquaculture activity, including shrimp and salmon farming, potential damage to ocean and coastal resources through habitat destruction, waste disposal, exotic species and pathogen invasions, and large fish meal and fish oil requirements may further deplete wild fisheries stocks."[6]

This strong statement underscores the paradox—aquaculture was developed as a solution, but the practice has negatively affected wild fish populations and ocean health. Here's why: Farmed fish are fed a diet of fish oil and fish meal, which is manufactured from fish waste products and smaller fish (called forage fish) that are caught in the wild. This further depletes the wild fish population at a time when 75 percent of the world's monitored fisheries are already near or exceeding maximum sustainable yields.[7] These facts disprove a common misconception among fish consumers: they are not protecting wild fish when they choose farmed fish. (See chapter 6 to learn why farmed fish are not a safer, more healthful choice in the human diet.)

The authors of a study published in a September 2009 edition of the *Proceedings of the National Academy of Sciences* reported that fully one-third of the global wild fish catch goes to produce fish meal and fish oil for use in the fish-farming industry and for other agricultural purposes.[8] Nearly 60 percent of the fish meal produced in the world is used in Asia, mostly in China. These rising demands for wild fish to feed farmed fish "places direct pressure on fisheries resources," observed the authors of the *Nature* article.[9]

According to the *World Review of Fisheries and Aquaculture 2008*, more than half of the fish oil produced in the entire world is fed to farmed salmon.[10] As discussed in chapter 5, even the most health-conscious consumers don't realize that marine algae is the original source of omega-3 fatty acids. That's why herring and sardines, and other forage fish that eat algae and fish oil, are fed to farmed salmon.

The loss of wild fish populations cannot be attributed only to the practice of feeding wild fish, fish meal, and fish oil to farmed fish. An article in the November 2001 issue of *EMBO Reports*, the journal of the European Molecular Biology Organization, stated: "Most of the ocean fishing catch is simply discarded. . . . When analyzing a five-year survey of trawling operations in the Gulf of Mexico, it was found that only 16 percent of the total catch was commercially viable shrimp, while 68 percent of the total catch was unintended bycatch, mostly juvenile finfish. In some areas of the Gulf of Mexico, it is estimated that for every one kilogram of shrimp harvested, 10 kilograms of other species are caught and discarded."[11] Bycatch is the term the fishing industry uses to describe untargeted marine animals that happen to get caught. These fish are also dismissively called "trash fish."[12]

Stay Tuned for the Frankenfish Invasion

To solve the problem of overfishing and the diminishing populations of wild fish, scientists devised "Frankenfish"—genetically engineered (GE) fish that grow faster and bigger than normal fish. The first species to be modified was salmon.

Time magazine declared genetically modified North Atlantic salmon to be one of 2010's top fifty inventions because transgenic salmon, as they came to be known, were the first genetically modified animals intended for human consumption.[13] By some estimates, transgenic fish can grow to ten times the size of normal fish in the first year of life. This is accomplished by splicing a gene from a fish called ocean pout, which resembles an eel, into farm-raised Atlantic salmon. This process increases the amount of growth hormones and accelerates the salmon's natural growth cycle.

Most of the owners of the four thousand aquaculture facilities in the United States are applauding this innovation, as it means higher profits. AquaBounty Technologies, a company in New England, engineered the fish and filed an application with the US Food and Drug Administration (FDA) for approval. As of this writing, the FDA has yet to make a decision, but we can be fairly certain that transgenic fish will enter the marketplace eventually, whether in the United States or some other country.

The question we should be asking is this: what are the risks of contaminating the food supply with transgenic fish? Supporters of genetic modification argue that we are already surrounded by genetically modified food. Henry I. Miller, former director of the FDA's Office of Biotechnology, puts it this way: "Most of the corn, soy, and canola grown in the United States is genetically engineered with molecular techniques, and more than 80 percent of the processed food in our supermarkets contain ingredients from genetically engineered crops. In North America alone, consumers have eaten more than three trillion servings of food that contains ingredients from genetically engineered plants without a single documented adverse reaction."[14]

Animals are genetically manipulated for reasons beyond food production. Fans of genetic engineering do cartwheels of enthusiasm over such innovations as the GloFish, a zebra fish that is already on the market. This aquarium fish, which is marketed to hobbyists and beginners, has been genetically altered so that it glows fluorescently. Whether they are modified for food or just fun and games, have we overlooked some important considerations in our frenzy to manipulate living organisms?

Let's hear what a scientific expert believes about the risks of raising GE salmon in fish farms. Biologist Robert Devlin has studied these fish since 1989 on behalf of Fisheries and Oceans Canada, Center for Aquaculture and Environmental Research. He was interviewed by a newspaper reporter about his findings, and he made this observation: "There's still more questions than answers. It's complex. It's really puzzling. Simply put, we scientists can't say for sure how these fish will respond to different environments. There is a serious risk if they escape into the environment."[15]

Farmed salmon already routinely escape into the wild. "As much as 40 percent of Atlantic salmon caught by fishermen in areas of the North Atlantic Ocean are of farmed origin," reported a team of fisheries researchers in *Nature* back in June 2000.[16] They also stated: "In the North Pacific Ocean, over 255,000 Atlantic salmon have reportedly escaped since the early 1980s and are caught by fishing vessels from Washington to Alaska. Increasing evidence suggests that farm escapees may hybridize with and alter the genetic makeup of wild populations of Atlantic salmon that are genetically adapted to their natal spawning grounds. Such genetic alterations could exacerbate the decline in many locally endangered populations of wild Atlantic salmon."[17]

When GE salmon escape into the wild, they are capable of crowding out and eventually killing off natural species by inter-breeding and outcompeting them for food. According to estimates published in the *Proceedings of the National Academy of Sciences,* an escape of just sixty GE fish into a wild population of sixty thousand non-GE fish could lead to the extinction of the entire wild population within a matter of years.[18] Even though the company behind GE salmon insists the fish are sterile, biologists know that a certain percentage of fish will remain fertile and be able to reproduce in the wild. This possibility is enhanced because some fish can change their gender from male to female.

Authors of a study published in a November 2010 edition of *Science* urged the FDA to consider other threats from GE fish. They wrote: "Environmental concerns about salmon farming include local pollution from waste effluents, disease, and potentially increased pressure on wild fish stocks that provide sources of feed for salmon."[19]

For consumers, potential problems are the unknown health risks of eating GE fish and the task of trying to purchase unaffected fish. There may be no labeling of transgenic fish, making it impossible for people to identify them in supermarkets. Consumers simply won't have access to the information necessary to do so.

The company behind GE salmon adamantly opposes labeling transgenic fish, revealing its fear that consumers will choose non-GE fish if they are given a clear choice. Their opposition serves as an important reminder that, by manipulating nature, we raise many questions.

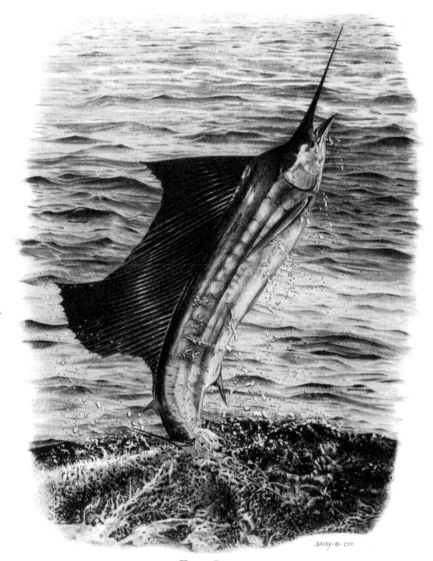

FREE JUMPER

CHAPTER EIGHT

All Sea Life May Perish in Our Lifetime

Whe the world's greatest marine scientists get together at international conferences, their primary topic of discussion, especially for the last five or so years, has been human actions that trigger and accelerate the decline of ocean habitats and species. During their April 2011 meeting at the University of Oxford, the scientists took these concerns about ocean health to a new level.

During this event organized by the International Programme on the State of the Ocean and the International Union for Conservation of Nature, these dozens of world science leaders came to conclusions that should be of concern to every human on the planet, but especially to people who continue to mindlessly eat fish and other ocean life. The scientists warn that we are experiencing severe declines in many species, to the point of commercial extinction, along with unparalleled rates of regional extinctions of habitat types. They say that we face losing—within a single generation—both marine species and the marine ecosystems on which they depend for survival.[1]

"If the various estimates we have received come true," remarked United Nations environmental official Pavan Sukhdev, "then we are in a situation where forty years down the line we, effectively, are out of fish." UN experts estimate that 30 percent of the world's fish stocks have already collapsed, and current trends project that virtually all of the fisheries in all of the oceans will be devoid of commercially viable catches by 2050.[2]

It's like a perfect ecological storm. As overfishing continues and humans eat some species to extinction, we see the combined effects of climate change, human-caused pollution, and habitat loss begin to produce a global extinction event in the ocean. What is happening in our oceans today is comparable to what happened when the dinosaurs and many other life-forms were extinguished. Scientists have documented that at least five global extinction events have occurred over the past 600 million years, and this latest one could rival them all.[3]

What's Gone Wrong

During the 2011 conference, the marine scientists uncovered several of the vital reasons sea life has reached this crisis. The following summarizes their major findings.[4]

Climate change. Habitat loss and overfishing are the primary causes of marine species extinction, but climate change is now playing a role in accelerating that process. Warmer water in the oceans forces some species into deeper, cooler waters, where they are unable to survive. Simultaneously, shifts in ocean currents, along with warmer temperatures caused by climate change, disrupt the food supplies of marine animals, further stressing the ability of entire species to adapt and survive in the altered climate.

Human activities. The extensive ecosystem damage caused by human actions is compromising the ocean's natural ability to adapt to climate change. Up to a certain point, the oceans display resilience when stressed by climate change, but human-caused disruptions have undermined that natural capacity to adapt. For instance, the combination of agricultural runoff and other pollutants, such as pathogens and endocrine-disrupting chemicals, has reduced the coral reefs' ability to recover. As a result, reef ecosystems are no longer dominated by coral but are dominated by algae, which hastens the loss of genetic diversity among fish and other ocean life.

Oxygen loss. Warming and acidification of the oceans, caused primarily by human actions, have accelerated the process of hypoxia. Hypoxia, which is detrimental to aerobic organisms, occurs when the amount of dissolved oxygen in a body of water is reduced. It doesn't take long before this oxygen deprivation sets in motion a chain reaction of die-off events, starting with microorganisms and then extending up the food chain.

Global outcomes. Many predicted worst-case scenarios about the ocean have already come to pass. There is a decrease in Arctic Sea ice, the Greenland ice sheet and the Antarctic ice sheets are melting, the sea level is rising, and more methane is being released from the world's sea beds. Such effects are compounding other problems, including the appearance of harmful algal blooms; the loss of large, long-lived fish species; and the overall destabilization of food webs in marine ecosystems.

The Deep Seas Are Overlooked

When we consider the effects of human activities on ocean life, we often forget the deepest waters, which are found at two hundred meters and below. This is the largest environment on the planet, making up about half of the Earth's surface, and for centuries it has been a dump site.

As part of an initiative called Census of Marine Life, marine scientists from numerous countries analyzed everything that humans now know about the deep-sea environment and the effects of human activities. The massive study results were released in August 2011.[5] The following findings about the deep seafloor—and the estimated 10 million species that live there—deserve to be factored into the discussion about whether it is justifiable to consume aquatic life.

Litter and waste. The routine dumping of certain types of waste from ships was banned by an international agreement in 1972. The practice persists, however, and an estimated 6.4 million tons of litter and waste from bulk carriers, tankers, fishing boats, and other sources are still dumped into deep seas annually. Almost all scientific surveys of the seafloor, which are done using remotely operated vehicles, detect waste products. The most common are plastics, aluminum cans, glass, metal, and fishing gear. "The impacts of litter on deep-sea habitats and fauna," reported the science team, "may include suffocation of animals from plastics, release of toxic chemicals, propagation of invasive species, [and] physical damage to sessile fauna such as cold-water corals from discarded trash."[6]

Sewage, dredge, and mining waste. One examined site, the deep water along the eastern US seaboard, is a dump for industrial and municipal waste such as raw sewage—an estimated 36 million tons of it. The waste contains high levels of persistent organic pollutants that produce "clear faunal changes at the seabed."[7] There has yet to be an adequate measure of contamination in the sea life that feeds on this fauna. Toxic mining waste is most commonly found in deep-sea areas near places like Papua New Guinea.

Pharmaceuticals. Until the 1980s, the island of Puerto Rico gave tax incentives to pharmaceutical companies that encouraged them to dump their waste materials into deep seas about forty miles north of the island. At least 387,000 tons of drug waste, which is equivalent to about 880 Boeing 747 airliners filled with toxins, were deposited in that area. "Studies of the region used for waste disposal found demonstrable changes in the marine microbial community," the science team wrote, "and these wastes were acutely toxic to many marine invertebrates."[8]

This sort of drug waste dumping has been occurring all over the planet. Antibiotics, antidepressants, birth control pills, cancer treatments, painkillers, and a host of other pharmaceutical waste materials are known to bioaccumulate up the food chain. In addition to the intentional dumping of expired medicines, drug residues enter the oceans as a result of human excretions into sewage systems.

Radioactive waste. Residue from weapons testing and even radioactive medical waste has been concentrated on the slope and canyons of the northeastern Atlantic Ocean, and smaller disposals have occurred in the northwestern Atlantic and the northeastern and northwestern Pacific Oceans. Most of this waste was stored in drums and tipped over the side of ships. Another source of high-level radioactive waste is sunken nuclear submarines, which represent a significant threat to the environment.

Industrial chemicals. The most commonly detected industrial toxins are persistent organic pollutants, such as dioxins, toxic metals, pesticides, herbicides, and plastics that are resistant to degradation and accumulate in deep-sea sediments. Contaminant levels in fish have only recently been measured. Initial findings show the presence of dioxins in red shrimp (*Aristeus antennatus*) in the western Mediterranean and in fish at depths of 900 to 1,500 meters in the northwestern Mediterranean. Bioaccumulation of polycyclic aromatic hydrocarbons in aquatic life is also being recorded in the deep Gulf of Mexico.

Pollution decay from lost ships. Many thousands of ships have sunk over just the past century, and no one has a complete count to adequately assess the possible contamination issues. In World War II alone, during the battle of the Atlantic between the United States, Britain, and Germany, nearly four thousand military and merchant ships sank, often in the deepest waters. Many of these ships carried munitions that now provide a persistent source of toxic pollution and threatens ecosystems and aquatic life. Further endangering these life-forms are the chemical warfare agents that the navies of various countries intentionally dumped in every ocean during the twentieth century.

Deep-sea mining and oil and gas exploration. Mining operations target manganese nodules, which grow on the deep seafloor over the course of millions of years. When these nodules are removed, local fauna becomes extinct. Other creatures are buried under layers of mining waste sediment, resulting in the extinction of even more life. "Large-scale mining activities have real potential to yield species extinction," reported the scientists.[9] Other mining targets include cobalt and polymetallic sulphides, which are built up by hydrothermal activity on the seafloor, mostly in the Pacific Ocean.

Oil and gas drilling now commonly occur at up to 3,000 meters of ocean depth. At such depths, the effects of accidents and incidental pollution are magnified. We need look no further than the April 2010 explosion at the Deepwater Horizon well in the Gulf of Mexico to see what happens when five million barrels of crude oil are released into the water. The environmental damage caused by that incident is still being seen and felt, and not just on beaches or surface waters. As reported in the November 5, 2010, *National Geographic News*, researchers have found colonies of coral covered with oil at 1,400 meters of depth, and this pollution has resulted in the corals' progressive death and the consequential extinction of aquatic life that depended on the coral.[10]

Human Activities Produce Many Microeffects

The studies and reports mentioned above were done at the macro level, and these findings are reinforced by information coming from observers at the micro level. For instance, consider what has been called "the great lobster die-off" in Long Island Sound, where nine-tenths of the lobster population disappeared over the past decade or so.

On August 8, 2011, the *New York Times* reported that the lobster has fallen victim to human actions: "Scientists blamed global warming, citing increased temperatures in the lower waters where lobsters live. Other culprits were pesticides like those deployed against the West Nile virus. The die-off began around the same time that the remnants of Hurricane Floyd swept over Long Island and, lobstermen believe, flushed pesticides into the Sound."[11]

Overfishing and the acidification of oceans (caused by rising concentrations of carbon dioxide in the atmosphere) create ideal conditions for explosions in the population of jellyfish. On July 8, 2011, a columnist for the *Guardian*, a British newspaper, reported that jellyfish had replaced mackerel as the predominant species in Cardigan Bay in west Wales. "Until 2010, mackerel were the one reliable catch in Cardigan Bay," wrote George Monbiot. "Last year it all changed. . . . Jellyfish. Unimaginable numbers of them. Not the transparent cocktail umbrellas I was used to, but solid, white rubbery creatures the size of footballs. They roiled in the surface or loomed, vast and pale, in the depths. There was scarcely a cubic meter of water without one."[12]

The week before Monbiot wrote his column, a monstrous swarm of jellyfish shut down both reactors at the Torness Nuclear Power Station in Scotland by clogging up the water-intake system. A few days later, another jellyfish swarm closed a nuclear power plant in Israel. Similar reports of jellyfish taking over otherwise empty ocean space have come in from all over the planet.[13]

Ocean acidification affects fish in yet another way that humans could have never predicted. On July 2, 2011, *Science News* reported that acidic water makes fish ear bones less dense, rendering some species of fish oblivious to alarming sounds. Because they are unable to distinguish the sounds of predators approaching, they become easier prey.

"Since the beginning of the Industrial Revolution," noted the article, "roughly 142 billion tons of human-made carbon dioxide has dissolved into the world's oceans. Adding the gas to seawater creates carbonic acid and is nudging water closer to the acidic end of the pH scale at the fastest pace in 650,000 years."[14]

Finally, consider what the warming and acidification of the ocean's waters is doing to fish migratory patterns. Since 2009, according to the *Telegraph*, a British newspaper, a fish that causes hallucinations when eaten has started to migrate into British waters from the Mediterranean and from off the coast of South Africa. It's a species of bream called *Sarpa salpa*, a plankton eater with golden stripes that poisons its predators with a hallucinogenic chemical. Humans who consume the fish can have vivid hallucinations that last for days. The newspaper recounted an incident involving two men in France (ages forty and ninety) who were hospitalized after eating *Sarpa salpa*. Within minutes after the meal, they experienced auditory hallucinations and nightmares that then lasted for several days.[15]

Our Introduction of Invasive Species Spreads Problems

Human attempts to tinker with ecosystems by introducing new fish species often backfire in unexpected ways that accelerate the decline of the planet's aquatic health. Consider what happened with the carp.

During the 1800s, fishermen in the midwestern United States introduced the common carp, native to other parts of the world, into the ecosystem, because this fish can grow to weigh dozens of pounds in muddy-bottomed lakes. In the 1960s, still other species of carp, such as the bighead and silver carp, were introduced into US ponds to eat the algae that had built up, mostly as a result of fertilizer runoff from agricultural lands.

As *Science News* reported on July 2, 2011, these species of carp have become invasive, crowding out other fish in the Mississippi and other river systems to near extinction. These carp can grow to one hundred pounds, every day eating up to 120 percent of their weight in plankton and algae, further depleting food sources for other species.[16]

Since 2010, city, state, and national governments have made desperate efforts to keep the carp from migrating upstream into the Great Lakes. The concern is that the carp will decimate the native fish populations in those bodies of water and catalyze the overall decline of ecosystems. Attempts have been made to stop the migration by erecting electrical underwater barriers at points where the lakes and river systems meet.[17] Given the escape record of these fish over the years, there is little reason to believe they won't end up invading the Great Lakes, once again demonstrating that nature, not humans, knows what is best for the natural balance of life.

Your Tax Dollars Accelerate Harm

Taxpayers in the United States and other countries contribute to overfishing and the decline of entire fish species because their governments provide large subsidies to the commercial fishing industry. In 2009 researchers with the Environmental Working Group (EWG) calculated that US taxpayers dole out nearly $1 billion each year in fishing subsidies from federal and state governments. The practice, EWG says, "is accelerating the ongoing collapse of fish stocks worldwide and adding to the devastation of large ocean fish species."[18]

Nearly half of US fishing subsidies cover fishing fleet fuel costs, according to the EWG. Unlike truckers and motorists, commercial fishing fleets remain exempt from all state and federal fuel taxes, which encourages the fishing companies to keep as many ships out to sea as possible. An analysis by the World Bank found that, on average, each ton of fish caught requires about half a ton of fuel.[19]

Nearly one-third of the 269 monitored fish stocks in US waters are overfished, according to National Marine Fishery Service records from 1997 onward. The global situation is comparable—there are too many fishing boats chasing a diminishing number of fish. So governments subsidize fishermen, primarily salmon and tuna fishermen.[20] Government policies like these should be among the first targets of those who work to bring about a change in global ecological consciousness.

Scientists Offer a List of Common-Sense Steps

The scientists attending the 2011 International Programme on the State of the Ocean put together a draft of recommendations for the governments of the world. They called for the following "urgent actions" to help restore the structure and function of marine ecosystems:

1. Reduce fishing to levels commensurate with long-term sustainability of fisheries and the marine environment.

2. Close fisheries that are not demonstrably managed following sustainable principles or that depend wholly on government subsidies.

3. Establish a globally comprehensive system of protected marine areas to conserve biodiversity, to build resilience, and to ensure ecologically sustainable fishing that leaves a minimal ecological footprint.

4. Prevent, reduce, and strictly control inputs into the marine environment of substances that are harmful or toxic to marine organisms.

5. Prevent, reduce, and strictly control nutrient inputs into the marine environment through better land and river catchment management and sewage treatment.

6. Avoid, reduce, or, at minimum, universally and stringently regulate oil, gas, aggregate, and mineral extraction from the oceans.

7. Properly and universally implement the precautionary principle by reversing the burden of proof so activities proceed only if they are shown not to harm the ocean singly or in combination with other activities.

Conclusion

I have long talked and written about positive and negative synergies when it comes to the human diet. Simply put, various nutrients interact to produce greater positive effects, and various synthetic chemicals and contaminants interact to magnify negative health consequences.

The same principles of synergy apply to aquatic ecosystems and the creatures that call them home. The threats discussed in this book, from industrial and consumer pollutants to overfishing, are compounded through synergy. As a result, fish and other aquatic life-forms have become contaminated and endangered. Their ability to reproduce has been compromised, and their genetics have been altered. The survival of entire species is at risk. It's not their fault, of course. Their health and habitats have been ruined exclusively by human actions.

As described in chapter 8, the world's leading marine scientists have proposed solutions to the current crisis in our oceans and waterways. These experts have issued an urgent call to action. Whether or not the world's governments and the fishing industry respond remains to be seen.

While these matters are being addressed at higher levels, we must thoughtfully evaluate our own actions. What we as individuals decide to do on behalf of aquatic life-forms and their plight is of the utmost importance, and I hope you will consider some possible alternatives and actions.

What matters to most people, of course, is whether or not fish and other sea animals are safe to eat. I maintain that they are not.

The toxins in fish work their way up the food chain, threatening the health of all people who consume fish and other seafood.

The fishing industry has a vested interest in concealing the dangers of eating fish, and government agencies have a poor track record of warning consumers or requiring informative labels. Therefore, it's virtually impossible to be an educated consumer and buy only the "safe" fish. Choosing farmed fish as an alternative to wild fish is certainly not a safe option. Farmed fish are fed a diet of fish meal and fish oil derived from wild fish, so they harbor all of the contaminants, including heavy metals, found in wild fish. In addition, farmed fish may be more likely to be infected with pathogens, including viruses, because the fish are confined together in great numbers.

Alternatives

Can you in good conscience slowly poison yourself—and by extension, contribute to the poisoning of the environment—by continuing to consume fish and related aquatic life? If your answer is no, I'd like to offer you some alternatives. For example, you can still get plenty of omega-3 fatty acids from other sources. These necessary nutrients are generated only by plants, and adequate amounts can be obtained by consuming marine algae (the same source fish obtain them from) and other plant-based foods, such as chia seeds, spinach, and walnuts.

You can also continue to enjoy the bounty of the seas, provided you substitute sea vegetables and blue-green algae, such as chlorella and spirulina, for fish. Marine algae is a veritable elixir for human health. Spirulina, for example, contains all of the essential amino acids, making it a source of complete protein. It also has thiamine, riboflavin, nicotinamide, pyridoxine, folic acid, and vitamins A, C, D, and E.

The second volume of my three-volume series of books, *Food IS Medicine: The Scientific Evidence,* contains dozens of peer-reviewed studies that reveal the medicinal value of eating certain aquatic plants. In *Edible Plant Foods, Fruits, and Spices from A to Z: Evidence for Their Healing Properties,* I identify dozens of health conditions that can either be treated or prevented by eating sea vegetables and marine algae. These include Alzheimer's disease, arterial disease, cancer, diabetes, fibromyalgia, high blood pressure, high cholesterol, irritable bowel syndrome, obesity, osteoporosis, Parkinson's disease, and many others.

Next Steps

I wrote this book because I am concerned about what is happening to the fish and their ecosystems. My professional focus, however, is on human health, and I believe your mental and physical health will be advanced by a vegetarian diet, free of fish. Better yet, go vegan and avoid all animal-based foods, including dairy products and eggs.

Vegetarians typically weigh up to twenty pounds less than meat eaters. Unlike harmful fad diets, which leave you feeling tired and inevitably fail as the weight returns, going vegetarian is the healthful way to keep the excess fat off for good, while keeping your energy level high.

According to the Academy of Nutrition and Dietetics, vegetarians are less likely to develop heart disease, cancer, diabetes, and high blood pressure than meat eaters. Vegetarians get all the nutrients they need to be healthy (vitamins, minerals, protein, and fiber) without consuming any of the contaminants and health-depleting fat and cholesterol in fish and other meat.

Your eating habits and buying decisions affect not only your health but also the lives of the animals you choose to eat—or not to eat. Every vegetarian helps prevent the horrific abuse inherent in modern animal agriculture, including fish farming. By choosing plant foods, every vegetarian saves more than one hundred animal lives each year. When you choose vegetarian foods over fish, meat, dairy products, and eggs, you make a statement that all life is important and has value—including your own.

Reference Notes

Introduction

1. Jane Allhouse, Jean Buzby, David Harvey et al., "International trade and seafood safety," *International Trade and Food Safety* AER-828 (2004): 109.

2. Jennifer Fisher Wilson, "Balancing the risks and benefits of fish consumption," *Ann Intern Med* 141, no. 2 (December 21, 2004): 977–80.

3. Jonathan Safran Foer, *Eating Animals* (New York: Little, Brown and Company, 2009).

Chapter One

1. Elizabeth Grossman, *Chasing Molecules: Poisonous Products, Human Health, and the Promise of Green Chemistry* (Washington, DC: Shearwater, 2009).

2. United Nations Environment Programme, "Stockholm Convention on Persistent Organic Pollutants," 2001, chm.pops.int/Convention/tabid/54/Default.aspx.

3. See note 1 above.

4. Spencer Peterson, John Van Sickle, Alan Herlihy et al., "Mercury concentrations in fish from streams and rivers throughout the western United States," *Environ Sci Technol* 41, no. 1 (2007): 58–65.

5. Chad Hammerschmidt and William Fitzerald, "Methylmercury in freshwater fish linked to atmospheric mercury deposition," *Environ Sci Technol* 40, no. 24 (2006): 7764–70.

6. W. Fitzgerald, D. Engstrom, R. Mason et al., "The case for atmospheric mercury contamination in remote areas," *Environ Sci Technol* 32, no. 1 (1998): 1–7.

7. S. P. Bhavsar et al., "Change in mercury levels in Great Lakes fish between 1970s and 2007," *Environ Sci Technol* 44, no. 9 (2010): 3273–9.

8. California Department of Health Services, *Research, Education, and Outreach on Fish Contamination in the Sacramento-San Joaquin Delta and Tributaries,* January 2004, ehib.org/papers/NeedsAssessmentDF.pdf.

9. California Environmental Protection Agency Office of Environmental Health Hazard Assessment, *OEHHA Issues Updated Fish Advisory for San Francisco Bay,* May 23, 2011, oehha.ca.gov/fish/nor_cal/pdf/SFBaypress052311.pdf.

10. US Food and Drug Administration, "Mercury levels in commercial fish and shellfish 1990-2010," fda.gov/Food/FoodSafety/Product-SpecificInformation/Seafood/FoodbornePathogensContaminants/Methylmercury/default.htm.

11. S. L. Gerstenberger and J. A. Dellinger, "PCBs, mercury, and organochlorine concentrations in lake trout, walleye, and whitefish from selected tribal fisheries in the Upper Great Lakes region," *Environ Toxicol* 17, no. 6 (2002): 513-9.

12. R. F. Pearson et al., "Concentrations, accumulations, and inventories of toxaphene in sediments of the Great Lakes," *Environ Sci Technol* 31, no. 12 (1997): 3523-9.

13. California Environmental Protection Agency Office of Environmental Health Hazard Assessment, *OEHHA Issues Fish Advisory for Donner Lake,* January 27, 2011, oehha.ca.gov/public_info/press/donnerpress012711.pdf.

14. M. S. Evans et al., "Persistent organic pollutants and metals in the freshwater biota of the Canadian Subarctic and Arctic: an overview," *Sci Total Environ* 351-2 (December 1, 2005): 94-147.

15. S. Hardell et al., "Levels of polychlorinated biphenyls (PCBs) and three organochlorine pesticides in fish from the Aleutian Islands of Alaska," *PLoS One* 5, no. 8 (August 25, 2010): e12396.

16. K. Arisawa et al., "Fish intake, plasma omega-3 polyunsaturated fatty acids, and polychlorinated dibenzo-p-dioxins/polychlorinated dibenzo-furans and co-planar polychlorinated biphenyls in the blood of the Japanese population," *Int Arch Occup Environ Health* 76, no. 3 (April 2003): 205-15.

17. S. Bayen et al., "Persistent organic pollutants and heavy metals in typical seafood consumed in Singapore," *Journal Toxicol Environ Health A* 68, no. 3 (February 13, 2005): 151-66.

18. A. Covaci et al., "Levels and distribution of organochlorine pesticides, polychlorinated biphenyls, and polybrominated diphenyl ethers in sediments and biota from the Danube Delta, Romania," *Environ Pollut* 140, no. 1 (March 2006): 136-49.

19. J. L. Domingo et al., "Human exposure to PBDEs through the diet in Catalonia, Spain: temporal trend. A review of recent literature on dietary PBDE intake," *Toxicology* 248, no. 1 (June 3, 2008): 25–32.

20. G. Falco et al., "Exposure to hexachlorobenzene through fish and seafood consumption in Catalonia, Spain," *Sci Total Environ* 389, nos. 2–3 (January 25, 2008): 289–95.

21. M. Perugini et al., "Polycyclic aromatic hydrocarbons in marine organisms from the Adriatic Sea, Italy," *Chemosphere* 66, no. 10 (January 2007): 1904–10.

22. P. Visciano et al., "Polycyclic aromatic hydrocarbons in farmed rainbow trout (*Oncorhynchus mykiss*) processed by traditional flue gas smoking and by liquid smoke flavourings," *Food Chem Toxicol* 46, no. 5 (May 2008): 1409–13.

23. P. Visciano et al., "Polycyclic aromatic hydrocarbons in fresh and cold-smoked Atlantic salmon fillets," *J Food Prot* 69, no. 5 (May 2006): 1134–8.

24. J. M. Liobet et al., "Exposure to polycyclic aromatic hydrocarbons through consumption of edible marine species in Catalonia, Spain," *J Food Prot* 69, no. 10 (October 2006): 2493–9.

25. L. Duedahl-Olesen et al., "Influence of smoking parameters on the concentration of polycyclic aromatic hydrocarbons (PAHs) in Danish smoked fish," *Food Addit Contam Part A* 27, no. 9 (September 2010): 1294–305.

26. M. M. Storelli et al., "Polycyclic aromatic hydrocarbons in mussels (*Mytilus galloprovincialis*) from the Ionian Sea, Italy," *J Food Prot* 64, no. 3 (March 2001): 405–9.

27. See note 15 above.

28. J. E. Hinck et al., "Chemical contaminants, health indicators, and reproductive biomarker responses in fish from rivers in the southeastern United States," *Sci Total Environ* 390, nos. 2–3 (February 15, 2008): 538–57.

29. J. E. Hinck et al., "Chemical contaminants, health indicators, and reproductive biomarker responses in fish from the Colorado River and its tributaries," *Sci Total Environ* 378, no. 3 (June 1, 2007): 376–402.

30. J. E. Hinck et al., "Widespread occurrence of intersex in black basses (*Micropterus spp.*) from US rivers, 1995–2004," *Aquat Toxicol* 95, no. 1 (October 19, 2009): 60–70.

31. Florida Department of Health, "Fish consumption advisories," myflori-daeh.com/medicine/fishconsumptionadvisories.

32. Fen Montaigne, "Still waters, the global fish crisis," *National Geographic*, April 2007, ngm.nationalgeographic.com/2007/04/global-fisheries-crisis/montaigne-text.

33. Daniel J. Madigan, Zofia Baumann, and Nicholas S. Fisher, "Pacific bluefin tuna transport Fukushima-derived radionuclides from Japan to California," *P Natal Aca Sci USA*, May 29, 2012 (Epub ahead of print).

34. Alicia Chang, "Radioactive bluefin tuna: Japan nuclear plant contaminated fish found off California coast," *Huffington Post*, May 28, 2012.

35. Cain Burdeau, "Two years after BP oil spill, sick fish found in gulf," *Associated Press*, April 19, 2012.

Chapter Two

1. Jennifer Fisher Wilson, "Balancing the risks and benefits of fish consumption," *Ann Intern Med* 141, no. 2 (December 21, 2004): 977–80.

2. B. J. Wallace et al., "Seafood-associated disease outbreaks in New York, 1980–1994," *Am J Prev Med* 17, no. 1 (July 1999): 48–54.

3. J. Sumner et al., "A semiquantitative seafood safety risk assessment," *Int J Food Microbiol* 77, nos. 1–2 (July 25, 2002): 55–9.

4. J. Y. Ting and A. F. Brown, "Ciguatera poisoning: a global issue with common management problems," *Eur J Emerg Med* 8, no. 4 (December 2001): 295–300.

5. E. K. Lipp and J. B. Rose, "The role of seafood in foodborne diseases in the United States of America," *Rev Sci Tech* 16, no. 2 (August 1997): 620–40.

6. Roshini Raj, "What the yuck? Mercury poisoning from sushi?" *CNN Health*, April 8, 2011, thechart.blogs.cnn.com/2011/04/08/what-the-yuck-mercury-poisoning-from-sushi.

7. See note 6 above.

8. L. C. Chien, C. S. Gao, and H. H. Lin, "Hair mercury concentration and fish consumption: risk and perceptions of risk among women of childbearing age," *Environ Res* 110, no. 1 (January 2010): 123–9.

9. M. Sakamoto, M. Kubota, X. J. Liu et al., "Maternal and fetal mercury and n-3 polyunsaturated fatty acids as a risk and benefit of fish consumption to fetus," *Environ Sci Technol* 38, no. 14 (July 15, 2001): 3860–3.

10. S. Diez, S. Elgado, and I. Aguilera et al., "Prenatal and early childhood exposure to mercury and methylmercury in Spain, a high-fish-consumer country," *Arch Environ Contam Toxicol* 56, no. 3 (April 2009): 615–22.

11. K. A. Bjornberg, M. Vahter, K. P. Grawe et al., "Methylmercury exposure in Swedish women with high fish consumption," *Sci Total Environ* 342, nos. 1–3 (April 1, 2005): 45–52.

12. J. T. Salonen et al., "Intake of mercury from fish, lipid peroxidation, and the risk of myocardial infarction and coronary, cardiovascular, and any death in eastern Finnish men," *Circulation* 91, no. 3 (February 1,1995): 645–55.

13. J. K. Virtanen et al., "Mercury, fish oils, and risk of acute coronary events and cardiovascular disease, coronary heart disease, and all-cause mortality in men in eastern Finland," *Arterioscler Thromb Vasc Biol* 25, no. 1 (January 2005): 228–33.

14. Marian Burros, "High mercury levels are found in tuna sushi," *New York Times,* January 23, 2008.

15. D. H. Phillips, "Polycyclic aromatic hydrocarbons in the diet," *Mutat Res* 443, nos. 1–2 (July 15, 1999): 139–47.

16. J. M. Liobet, G. Falco, A. Bocio et al., "Exposure to polycyclic aromatic hydrocarbons through consumption of edible marine species in Catalonia, Spain," *J Food Prot* 69, no. 10 (October): 2493–9.

17. P. Visciano, M. Perugini, M. Amoerena et al., "Polycylic aromatic hydrocarbons in fresh and cold-smoked Atlantic salmon fillets," *J Food Prot* 69, no. 5 (May 2006): 1134–8.

18. David O. Carpenter, "Polychlorinated biphenyls (PCBs): routes of exposure and effects on human health," *Rev Environ Health* 21, no. 1 (January–March 2006): 1–23.

19. S. L. Schantz et al., "Impairments of memory and learning in older adults exposed to polychlorinated biphenyls via consumption of Great Lakes fish," *Environ Health Persp* 109, no. 5 (June 2001): 605.

20. N. Codru et al., "Diabetes in relation to serum levels of polychlorinated biphenyls and chlorinated pesticides in adult Native Americans," *Environ Health Persp* 115, no. 10 (October 2007): 1442–7.

21. A. Goncharov, "High serum PCBs are associated with elevation of serum lipids and cardiovascular disease in a Native American population," *Environ Res* 106, no. 2 (February 2008): 226–39.

22. X. Huang et al., "Consumption advisories from salmon based on risk of cancer and noncancerous health effects," *Environ Res* 101, no. 2 (June 2006): 263–74.

23. See note 22 above.

24. A. Bocio, J. M. Llobet, J. L. Domingo et al., "Polybrominated diphenyl ethers (PBDEs) in foodstuffs: human exposure through diet," *J Agric Food Chem* 51, no. 10 (2003): 3191–5.

25. S. Bayen et al., "Persistent organic pollutants and heavy metals in typical seafoods consumed in Singapore," *J Toxic Env Health A* 68, no. 3 (February 13, 2005): 151–66.

26. Kathleen McAuliffe, "There's something in the water," *Discover*, May 2011, 41–6.

27. See note 26 above.

28. See note 26 above.

Chapter Three

1. I. S. Shin et al., "Bactericidal activity of wasabi (*Wasabia japonica*) against *Helicobacter pylori*," *Int J Food Microbiol* 94, no. 3 (August 1, 2004): 255–61.

2. Marian Burros, "High mercury levels are found in tuna sushi," *New York Times*, January 23, 2008.

3. See note 2 above.

4. See note 2 above.

5. "Sushi eaters weigh the health risks," *New York Times*, January 23, 2008.

6. J. H. Lowenstein et al., "DNA barcodes reveal species-specific mercury levels in tuna sushi that pose a health risk to consumers," *Biology Letters* 6, no. 5 (October 23, 2010): 692–5.

7. See note 6 above.

8. Danny Penman, "Sushi—the raw truth," *Daily Mail,* April 4, 2006.

9. See note 8 above.

10. David O. Carpenter et al., "Benefits versus risks associated with consumption of fish and other seafood," *Rev Environ Health* 25, no. 3 (2010): 161–91.

11. S. D. Shaw et al., "Polybrominated diphenyl ethers (PBDEs) in farmed and wild salmon marketed in the northeastern United States," *Chemosphere* 71, no. 8 (April 2008): 1422–31.

12. V. Atanassova, F. Reich, and G. Klein, "Microbiological quality of sushi from sushi bars and retailers," *J Food Prot* 71, no. 4 (April 2008): 860–4.

13. J. Barralet, R. Stafford, C. Towner et al., "Outbreak of *Salmonella singapore* associated with eating sushi," *Commun Dis Intell* 28, no. 4 (2004): 527–8.

14. See note 13 above.

15. J. Suzuki et al., "Risk factors for human Anisakis infection and association between the geographic origins of *Scomber japonicas* and anisakid nematodes," *Int J Food Microbiol* 137, no. 1 (January 31, 2010): 88–93.

Chapter Four

1. E. Gray et al., "Latent effects of pesticides and toxic substances on sexual differentiation of rodents," *Toxicol Ind Health* 12, nos. 3–4 (May 1996): 515–531.

2. Nicholas D. Kristof, "It's time to learn from frogs," *New York Times,* June 27, 2009.

3. B. W. Brooks et al., "Occurrence of pharmaceuticals and personal care products in fish: Results of a national pilot study in the United States," *Environ Toxicol Chem* 28, no. 12 (December 2009): 2587–97.

4. S. Sauvé et al., "Distribution of antidepressants and their metabolites in brook trout exposed to municipal wastewaters before and after ozone treatment—evidence of biological effects," *Chemosphere* 83, no. 4 (April 2011): 564–71.

5. US Geological Survey, *Summary of US Geological Survey Information Related to the Intersex Characteristics of Fish in the Potomac Watershed,* accessed February 10, 2012, chesapeake.usgs.gov/feature/fishhealthWW-Wfeature.pdf.

6. David Fahrenthold, "Male bass across region found to be bearing eggs," *Washington Post,* September 6, 2006, A1.

7. Michael Rollins, "A medicine cabinet runs through it," *Portland Oregonian,* March 10, 2008.

8. See note 7 above.

9. Z. Zhang and J. Hu, "Effects of p,p'-DDE exposure on gonadal development and gene expression in Japanese medaka (*Oryzias latipes*)," *J Environ Sci* 20, no. 3 (2008): 347–52.

10. J. G. Vos et al., "Health effects of endocrine-disrupting chemicals on wildlife, with special reference to the European situation," *Crit Rev Toxicol* 30, no. 2 (January 2000): 71–133.

11. M. A. Kelly et al., "Investigation of the estrogenic risk to feral male brown trout (*Salmo trutta*) in the Shannon International River Basin District of Ireland," *Ecotoxicol Environ Saf* 73, no. 7 (October 2010): 1658–65.

12. A. Mandich et al., "In vivo exposure of carp to graded concentrations of bisphenol A," *Gen Comp Endocrinol* 153, nos. 1–3 (August–September 2007): 15–24.

13. A. P. Scott et al., "Evidence for estrogenic endocrine disruption in an offshore flatfish, the dab (*Limanda limando L.*)," *Marine Environ Res* 64, no. 2 (August 2007): 128–48.

14. I. E. Barnhoorn et al., "Intersex in feral indigenous freshwater *Oreochromis mossambicus*, from various parts in the Luvuvhu River, Limpopo Province, South Africa," *Ectotoxicol Environ Saf* 73, no. 7 (October 2010): 1537–42.

15. K. A. Kidd et al., "Collapse of a fish population after exposure to a synthetic estrogen," *P Natl Acad of Sci* 104, no. 21 (May 22, 2007): 8897–901.

16. John Roach, "Sex-changing chemicals can wipe out fish, study shows," *National Geographic News,* May 21, 2007.

17. B. S. Chesman, "Intersex in the clam *Scrobicularia plana*: a sign of endocrine disruption in estuaries?" *Biological Letters* 2, no. 3 (September 22, 2006): 420–2.

18. M. J. Bebianno, "Polycyclic aromatic hydrocarbons concentrations and biomarker responses in the clam *Ruditapes decussatus* transplanted in the Ria Formosa Lagoon," *Ecotox Environ Safe* 72, no. 7 (October 2009): 1849–60.

19. Randall Fitzgerald, *The Hundred Year Lie: How Food and Medicine Are Destroying Your Health* (New York: Penguin/Dutton, 2006).

20. Samuel J. Epstein, *Toxic Beauty* (Dallas: BenBella, 2008).

21. D. Schlenk et al., "In vivo bioassay-guided fractionation of marine sediment extracts from the Southern California Bight for estrogenic activity," *Environ Toxicol Chem* 24, no. 11 (November 2005): 2820–6.

22. M. E. Balmer, "Occurrence of some organic UV filters in wastewater, in surface waters, and in fish from Swiss lakes," *Environ Sci Technol* 39, no. 4 (February 15, 2005): 953–62.

23. A. M. Vajda et al., "Reproductive disruption in fish downstream from an estrogenic wastewater effluent," *Environ Sci Technol* 42, no. 9 (May 1, 2008): 3407–14.

24. C. Staples, U. Friedrich, H. Tilghman et al., "Estimating potential risks to terrestrial invertebrates and plants exposed to bisphenol A in soil amended with activated sludge biosolids," *Environ Toxicol Chem* 29, no. 2 (February 2010): 467–75.

25. L. B. Bjerregaard et al., "Sex hormone concentrations and gonad histology in brown trout (*Salmo trutta*) exposed to 17beta-estradiol and bisphenol A," *Ecotoxicology* 17, no. 4 (May 2008): 252–63.

26. A. Lange et al., "Sexual reprogramming and estrogenic sensitization in wild fish exposed to ethinylestradiol," *Environ Sci Technol* 43, no. 4 (February 15, 2009): 1219–25.

27. S. Jobling et al., "Predicted exposures to steroid estrogens in UK rivers correlate with widespread sexual disruption in wild fish populations," *Environ Health Perspect* 114, supplement 1 (April 2006): 32–9.

28. J. W. Kwon et al., "Determination of 17alpha-ethynylestradiol, carbamazepine, diazepam, simvastatin, and oxybenzone in fish livers," *J AOAC Int* 92, no. 1 (January–February 2009): 359–69.

29. J. E. Hinck et al., "Chemical contaminants, health indicators, and reproductive biomarker responses in fish from rivers in the southeastern United States," *Sci Total Environ* 390, nos. 2–3 (February 15, 2008): 538–57.

30. J. E. Hinck et al., "Chemical contaminants, health indicators, and reproductive biomarker responses in fish from the Colorado River and its tributaries," *Sci Total Environ* 378, no. 3 (June 1, 2007): 378–402.

31. J. C. Fournier et al., "Antidepressant drug effects and depression severity," *J Amer Med Assoc* 303, no. 1 (2010): 47–53.

32. B. W. Brooks et al., "Determination of select antidepressants in fish from an effluent-dominated stream," *Environ Toxicol Chem* 24, no. 2 (February 2005): 464–9.

33. S. Chu and C. D. Metcalfe, "Analysis of paroxetine, fluoxetine, and norfluoxetine in fish tissues using pressurized liquid extraction, mixed mode solid phase extraction cleanup, and liquid chromatography-tandem mass spectrometry," *J Chromatogr A* 1163, nos. 1–2 (September 7, 2007): 112–8.

34. See note 3 above.

Chapter Five

1. P. Pietinen et al., "Intake of fatty acids and risk of coronary heart disease in a cohort of Finnish men: the alpha-tocopherol, beta-carotene cancer prevention study," *Am J Epidemiol* 145, no. 10 (1997): 876–87.

2. L. M. Arterburn et al., "Algal-oil capsules and cooked salmon: nutritionally equivalent sources of docosahexaenoic acid," *J Am Diet Assoc* 108, no. 7 (July 2008): 1204–9.

3. K. L. Weaver et al., "The content of favorable and unfavorable polyunsaturated fatty acids found in commonly eaten fish," *J Am Diet Assoc* 108, no. 7 (July 2008): 1178–85.

4. "Popular fish, tilapia, contains potentially dangerous fatty acid combination," *Science Daily*, July 8, 2008, sciencedaily.com/releases/2008/07/080708092228.htm.

5. See note 3 above.

6. H. L. Woodworth et al., "Dietary fish oil alters T lymphocyte cell populations and exacerbates disease in a mouse model of inflammatory colitis," *Cancer Research* 7, no. 20 (October 15, 2010): 7960–9.

7. "Fish oil linked to increased risk of colon cancer in mice," *Science Daily*, October 6, 2010, sciencedaily.com/releases/2010/10/101005104342.htm.

8. J. Delarue et al., "Fish oil supplementation reduces stimulation of plasma glucose fluxes during exercise in untrained males," *Brit J Nutr* 90 (2003): 777–86.

9. R. A. Gibson et al., "Effect of DHA supplementation during pregnancy on maternal depression and neurodevelopment of young children: a randomized controlled trial," *J Am Med Assoc* 304, no. 15 (October 20, 2010): 1675–83.

10. J. F. Quinn et al., "Docosahexaenoic acid supplementation and cognitive decline in Alzheimer's disease: a randomized trial," *J Amer Med Assoc* 304, no. 17 (November 3, 2010): 1903–11.

11. See note 10 above.

12. L. Harbige, "Fatty acids, the immune response, and autoimmunity: a question of n-6 essentiality and the balance between n-6 and n-3," *Lipids* 38, no. 4 (2003): 323–41.

13. L. Hooper et al., "Risks and benefits of omega-3 fats for mortality, cardiovascular disease, and cancer: systematic review," *Brit Med J* 323 (2006): 752.

14. T. Mori et al., "Omega-3 fatty acids and inflammation," *Cur Atheroscler Rep* 6, no. 6 (2004): 461–7.

15. "Women with type 1 diabetes receive no heart benefit from omega 3," *Medical News Today,* June 28, 2010, medicalnewstoday.com/articles/193107.php.

16. P. Angerer et al., "Effect of dietary supplementation with omega-3 fatty acids on progression of atherosclerosis in carotid arteries," *Cardiovasc Res* 54 (2002): 183–90.

17. C. Von Schacky et al., "The effect of dietary omega-3 fatty acids on coronary atherosclerosis: a randomized double-blind, placebo-controlled trial," *Ann Intern Med* 130, no. 7 (April 6, 1999): 554–62.

18. A. Ascherio et al., "Dietary intake of marine n-3 fatty acids, fish intake, and the risk of coronary disease among men," *New Engl J Med* 332, no. 15 (April 13, 1995): 977–82.

19. M. L. Burr et al., "Lack of benefit of dietary advice to men with angina: results of a controlled trial," *Eur J Clin Nutr* 57, no. 2 (February 2003): 193–200.

20. Brian Peskin, "Warning: fish oil contains no true EFAS—physicians may be unknowingly prescribing the wrong substance to patients causing great harm—PEOS solve this problem," *Explore* 19, no. 6 (2010).

21. See note 20 above.

22. Robert Rowen, "Is this the most controversial stance I've ever taken?" *Second Opinion* 21, no. 6 (June 2011).

23. See note 22 above.

24. See note 22 above.

25. S. H. Lee, H. J. Kang, H. J. Lee et al., "Six-week supplementation with chlorella has favorable impact on antioxidant status in Korean male smokers," *Nutrition,* August 4, 2009 (Epub ahead of print).

26. M. A. Juarez-Oropeza, D. Mascher, P. V. Torres-Duran et al., "Effects of dietary spirulina on vascular reactivity," *J Med Food* 12, no. 1 (February 2009): 15–20.

27. P. Parikh, U. Mani, and U. Iyer, "Role of spirulina in the control of glycemia and lipidemia in type 2 diabetes mellitus," *J Med Food* 4, no. 4 (Winter 2001): 193–9.

28. H. J. Park, Y. J. Lee, H. K. Ryu et al., "A randomized double-blind, placebo-controlled study to establish the effects of spirulina in elderly Koreans," *Ann Nutr Metab* 53, no. 4 (2008): 322–8.

29. R. Manoukian, M. Citton, P. Huerta et al., "The effects of the blue-green algae *A. phanizomenon* flos-aquae on human natural killer cells," *IBC Library Series* 1911, chapter 3.1 (1998).

30. J. A. Joseph, B. Shukitt-Hale, N. A. Denisova et al., "Long-term dietary strawberry, spinach, or vitamin E supplementation retards the onset of age-related neuronal signal-transduction and cognitive behavioral deficits," *J Neurosci* 18, no. 19 (October 1, 1998): 8047–55.

31. M. Sarawat, P. Muthenna, P. Suryanarayana et al., "Dietary sources of aldose reductase inhibitors: prospects for alleviating diabetic complications," *Asia Pac J Clin Nutr* 17, no. 4 (2008): 558–65.

32. K. Matsubara, H. Matsumoto, Y. Mizushina et al., "Inhibitory effect of glycolipids from spinach on in vitro and ex vivo angiogenesis," *Oncol Rep* 14, no. 1 (July 2005): 157–60.

33. L. C. Tapsell, M. J. Batterham, G. Teuss et al., "Long-term effects of increased dietary polyunsaturated fat from walnuts on metabolic parameters in type II diabetes," *Eur J Clin Nutr* 63, no. 8 (August 2009): 1008–15.

34. T. L. Psota, S. K. Gebauer, and P. Kris-Etherton, "Dietary omega-3 fatty acid intake and cardiovascular disease," *Am J Cardiol* 98, no. 4A (August 21, 2006): 3i–18i.

35. A. Chisholm, J. Mann, M. Skeaff et al., "A diet rich in walnuts favourably influences plasma fatty acid profile in moderately hyperlipidaemic subjects," *Eur J Clin Nutr* 52, no. 1 (January 1998): 12–6.

36. W. E. Hardman and G. Ion, "Suppression of implanted MDA-MB 231 human breast cancer growth in nude mice by dietary walnut," *Nutr Cancer* 60, no. 5 (2008): 666–74.

Chapter Six

1. R. A. Hites et al., "Global assessment of organic contaminants in farmed salmon," *Science* 303, no. 5655 (January 9, 2004): 226–9.

2. See note 1 above.

3. New York University of Albany, Institute for Health and the Environment, *First Global Study Reveals Health Risks of Widely Eaten Farm-Raised Salmon,* albany.edu/ihe/salmonstudy/pressrelease.html.

4. See note 3 above.

5. R. L. Naylor, R. J. Goldburg, J. H. Primavera et al., "Effect of aquaculture on world fish supplies," *Nature* 405 (June 2000): 1017–24.

6. See note 3 above.

7. See note 5 above.

8. See note 5 above.

9. R. L. Naylor, R. W. Hardy, D. P. Bureau et al., "Feeding aquaculture in an era of finite resources," *P Natl Acad Sci,* 106, no. 96 (September 8, 2009): 15103–10.

10. National Oceanic and Atmospheric Administration, "Aquaculture in the United States," nmfs.noaa.gov/aquaculture/aquaculture_in_us.html.

11. Juliet Eilperin, "Fish farming's bounty isn't without barbs," *Washington Post,* January 24, 2005.

12. Fisheries and Aquaculture Department, Food and Agriculture Organization of the United Nations, *The State of World Fisheries and Aquaculture,* 2004, fao.org/DOCREP/007/y5600e/y5600e00.htm.

13. D. W. Cole, R. Cole, S. J. Gaydos et al., "Aquaculture: environmental, toxicological, and health issues," *Int J Hyg Environ Heal* 212 (2009): 369–77.

14. See note 13 above.

15. J. A. Foran, R. A. Hites, D. O. Carpenter et al., "A survey of metals in tissues of farmed Atlantic and wild Pacific salmon," *Environ Toxicol Chem* 23, no. 9 (September 2004): 2108–10.

16. S. D. Shaw, D. Brenner, M. L. Berger et al., "PCBs, PCDD/Fs, and organochlorine pesticides in farmed Atlantic salmon from Maine, eastern Canada, and Norway, and wild salmon from Alaska," *Environ Sci Tech* 40, no. 17 (September 1, 2006): 5347–54.

17. See note 13 above.

18. J. A. Foran et al., "Risk-based consumption advice for farmed Atlantic and wild Pacific salmon contaminated with dioxins and dioxin-like compounds," *Environ Health Persp* 113, no. 5 (May 2005): 552–6.

19. See note 18 above.

20. See note 18 above.

21. X. Huang et al., "Consumption advisories for salmon based on risk of cancer and noncancer health effects," *Environ Res* 101, no. 2 (June 2006): 263–74.

22. See note 21 above.

23. See note 1 above.

24. See note 21 above.

25. See note 18 above.

Chapter Seven

1. Fen Montaigne, "Still waters, the global fish crisis," *National Geographic,*

April 2007, ngm.nationalgeographic.com/2007/04/global-fisheries-crisis/montaigne-text.

2. See note 1 above.

3. B. Worm et al., "Impacts of biodiversity loss on ocean ecosystem services," *Science* 314, no. 5800 (November 3, 2006): 787–90.

4. R. L. Naylor et al., "Effect of aquaculture on world fish supplies," *Nature* 405 (June 29, 2000): 1017–24.

5. R. W. Hardy et al., "Feeding aquaculture in an era of finite resources," *P Natal Aca Sci USA* 106, no. 96 (September 8, 2009): 15103–10.

6. See note 4 above.

7. Fisheries and Aquaculture Department, Food and Agriculture Organization of the United Nations, *The State of the World Fisheries and Aquaculture*, 2006, fao.org/fishery/sofia/en.

8. See note 5 above.

9. See note 4 above.

10. Fisheries and Aquaculture Department, Food and Agriculture Organization of the United Nations, *World Review of Fisheries and Aquaculture*, 2008 ftp://ftp.fao.org/docrep/fao/011/i0250e/i0250e01.pdf.

11. J. H. Tidwell et al., "Fish as food: aquaculture's contribution," *EMBO Reports* 2, no. 11 (November 15, 2001): 958–63.

12. See note 11 above.

13. Bryan Walsh, "Faster-growing salmon," *Time,* November 11, 2010.

14. Henry I. Miller, "Frankenfish fatuity," The Rationalist, *Forbes,* March 23, 2011, forbes.com/sites/henrymiller/2011/03/23/frankenfish-fatuity.

15. Tessa Holloway, "The science of bigger salmon," *North Shore News* (British Columbia), March 25, 2011, nsnews.com/health/story.html?id=4502286.

16. See note 4 above.

17. See note 4 above.

18. W. M. Muir and R. D. Howard, "Possible ecological risks of transgenic

organism release when transgenes affect mating success," *P Natal Aca Sci USA* 96 (1999): 13853–6.

19. M. D. Smith et al., "Genetically modified salmon and full impact assessment," *Science* 330 (November 19, 2010): 1052–3.

Chapter Eight

1. P. A. Tyler et al., "Man and the last great wilderness: human impact on the deep sea," *PLoS One* 6, no. 8 (August 1, 2011): e22588.

2. "Ocean's fish could disappear by 2050," *Discovery News*, May 17, 2010, news.discovery.com/earth/oceans-fish-fishing-industry.html.

3. A. D. Barnosky, N. Matzke, S. Tomiya et al., "Has the earth's sixth mass extinction already arrived?" *Nature* 471 (March 3, 2011): 51–7.

4. International Programme on the State of the Ocean, *Summary Report: International Earth System Expert Workshop on Ocean Stresses and Impacts*, June 21, 2011, stateoftheocean.org/pdfs/1806_IPSOshort.pdf.

5. See note 1 above.

6. See note 1 above.

7. See note 1 above.

8. See note 1 above.

9. See note 1 above.

10. Kathleen Jones, "Giant coral die-off found—gulf spill 'smoking gun?'" *National Geographic News*, November 5, 2010.

11. Barton Silverman and Michael Wilson, "The last of the lobstermen, chasing a vanishing treasure," *New York Times*, August 8, 2011, A12.

12. George Monbiot, "Have jellyfish come to rule the waves?' *The Guardian*, July 8, 2011.

13. See note 12 above.

14. Susan Millus, "Be more afraid, young clownfish," *Science News*, July 2, 2011, 12.

15. "Fish that triggers hallucinations found off British coast," *The Telegraph*, May 13, 2009, telegraph.co.uk/earth/earthnews/5318202/Fish-that-triggers-hallucinations-found-off-British-coast.html.

16. Elizabeth Quill, "A new carp comes to town," *Science News*, July 2, 2011, 32.

17. See note 16 above.

18. Environmental Working Group, "On the hook: commercial fishing reaps billions," March 2009, ewg.org/fishing-subsidies.

19. American Association for the Advancement of Science, "Session 2050: Will there be fish in the ocean?" Feb. 18, 2011, aaas.confex.com/aaas/2011/webprogram/Session 2904.html.

20. National Oceanic and Atmospheric Administration, *Catch Share Programs*, September 2009, noaa.gov/factsheets/new version/catch_shares.pdf.

21. See note 4 above.

Appendix: Scientific Case Studies Against Eating Fish

Cancer from Fish Consumption

"Cured meat, vegetables, and bean-curd foods in relation to childhood acute leukemia risk: a population based case-control study." C. Y. Liu, Y. H. Hsu, M. T. Wu et al. *BMC Cancer*. 2009 Jan 13;9:15. Key finding: "Consumption of cured/smoked meat and fish leads to the formation of carcinogenic N-nitroso compounds in the acidic stomach. A population-based case-control study was conducted of persons between 2 and 20 years old consisting of 145 acute leukemia cases and 370 age- and sex-matched controls. Consumption of cured/smoked meat and fish more than once a week was associated with an increased risk of acute leukemia, perhaps through their contents of nitrites and nitrosamines, while intake of vegetables . . . may be protective."

"Identification of a dietary pattern characterized by high-fat food choices associated with increased risk of breast cancer: the European Prospective Investigation into Cancer and Nutrition (EPIC)—Potsdam Study." M. Schulz, K. Hofmann, C. Weikert, U. Northlings, M. B. Schulze, and H. Boeing. *Br J Nutr*. 2008 Nov;100(5):942–6. Key finding: "Study participants were 15,351 female subjects free of cancer at baseline and with complete dietary and outcome information followed for an average of six years. We identified a food pattern characterized by high consumption of processed meat, fish, butter and other animal fats, and margarine explaining >42 percent of total variation in fatty acid intake. Adherence to this food pattern was associated with a two-fold risk of breast cancer. A food pattern characterized by high-fat food choices was significantly associated with increased risk of breast cancer."

"Foodstuffs and colorectal cancer risk: a review." P. Marques-Vidal, P. Ravasco, and M. Ermelinda Camilo. *Clin Nutr*. 2006 Feb;25(1):14–36. Key finding: "A systematic review of available prospective studies on dietary intake and colorectal cancer was conducted. Excessive consumption of meat or smoked/salted/processed food appears to be deleterious. The consumption of smoked or salted fish also increases risk for colorectal cancer. The consumption of white meat, fish/seafood, and dairy products was mostly unrelated to colorectal cancer risk."

"Exposure to polychlorinated biphenyls (PCBs) in food and cancer risk: recent advances." A. M. Roveda, L. Veronesi, R. Zoni, M. E. Colucci, and G. Sansebastiano. *Sanita Pubbl.* (Italian) 2006 Nov–Dec;62(6):677–96. Key finding: "Humans continue to be exposed to the toxic effects of PCBs because of their resistance to chemical and biological decomposition, their capacity of bioaccumulation, and their long half-life. Studies performed so far have pointed out a possible association between exposure to PCBs and increased risk of developing breast, prostate, testicular, ovarian, and uterine cancers. These compounds may also act as [endocrine disruptors] and cause infertility. PCBs accumulate in organisms through the food chain, and food accounts for 90 percent of exposure. The highest concentrations being found in fish (such as salmon and shellfish), dairy products (especially milk and butter), and animal fat."

"The influence of dietary patterns on the development of thyroid cancer." I. Markaki, D. Linos, and A. Linos. *Eur J Cancer.* 2003 Sep;39(13):1912–9. Key finding: "We conducted a case-control study of 113 persons with histologically verified thyroid cancer and 138 controls. Significant positive associations were observed for pork consumption. A dietary pattern of fish led to an increased risk of follicular cancer."

"Dietary factors and the risk of gastric cancer in Mexico City." M. H. Ward and L. Lopez-Carrillo. *Am J Epidemiol.* 1999 May 15;149(10):925–32. Key finding: "The authors conducted a population-based case-control study of gastric cancer in the Mexico City metropolitan area. A total of 220 patients with histologically confirmed gastric adenocarcinomas were interviewed and given a dietary questionnaire. There was approximately a threefold increased risk of gastric cancer for frequent consumption of both fresh meat and processed meat. Odds ratios were also significantly elevated for frequent consumption of dairy products and fish."

"Nutrition and lifestyle factors in fibrocystic disease and cancer of the breast." A. Simard, J. Vobecky, and J. S. Vobecky. *Cancer Detect Prev.* 1990;14(5):567–72. Key finding: "Within a study on diet as a risk factor for fibrocystic disease and breast cancer, 68 patients with breast cancer, aged from 40 to 59, participating in the National Breast Screening Study in Montreal, were compared to 340 patients with fibrocystic disease and to 343 controls. The cancer patients consumed significantly more poultry, fish, pastry, margarine, and alcohol."

Mercury Levels in Fish

"Hair mercury concentration and fish consumption: risk and perceptions of risk among women of childbearing age." L. C. Chien, C. S. Gao, and H. H. Lin. *Environ Res.* 2010 Jan;110(1):123–9. Key finding: "The purposes of this study were to assess the hair mercury concentration of women of childbearing age in Taiwan. The average concentration of mercury was 1.73+/-2.12microgg(-1), exceeding the US EPA reference dose of 1 microgg in 52.9 percent of study subjects. Hair mercury concentration in groups who consumed fish was significantly higher than in groups who never consumed fish."

"An evaluation of mercury concentrations in three brands of canned tuna." S. L. Gerstenberger, A. Martinson, and J. L. Kramer. *Environ Toxicol Chem.* 2010 Feb;29(2):237–42. Key finding: "In the present study, the amount of mercury present in canned tuna purchased in Las Vegas, Nevada, USA, was examined. Chunk white tuna and solid white tuna were both significantly higher in mercury than chunk light tuna. In total, 55 percent of all tuna examined was above the US EPA safety level for human consumption at 0.5 ppm. These results indicate that stricter regulation of the canned tuna industry is necessary to ensure the safety of sensitive populations such as pregnant women, infants, and children. According to the US EPA reference dose of 0.1 microg/kg body weight per day, a 25-kg child may consume a meal (75g) of canned chunk white tuna only once every 18.6 days."

"Mercury concentrations and omega-3 fatty acids in fish and shrimp: Preferential consumption for maximum health benefits." K. L. Smith and J. L. Guentzel. *Mar Pollut Bull.* 2010 Sep;60(9):1615–8. Key finding: "The consumption of fish and shrimp containing omega-3 fatty acids can result in protective health effects including a reduced risk of cardiovascular disease, stroke, and diabetes. These protective effects may be decreased by the presence of mercury in the muscle tissue of fish and shellfish. Mercury can increase the risk of cardiovascular problems and impede neurological development. The objective of this project was to determine appropriate consumption amounts of selected fish species and shrimp based on mercury levels and recommended intake levels of omega-3 fatty acids. Species that are high in omega-3s and low in mercury include salmon, trout, and shrimp. Species with both high levels of mercury and omega-3s include tuna, shark, halibut, swordfish, and sea bass."

"Hair mercury levels in pregnant women in Mahshahr, Iran: fish consumption as a determinant of exposure." Z. Salehi and A. Esmaili-Sari. *Sci Total Environ.* 2010 Sep 15;408(20):4848-54. Key finding: "149 pregnant women participated in this study. An interview administered questionnaire was used. The obtained results showed that the geometric mean and range for hair total mercury concentration was 3.52 microg/g. About 5.4 percent of mothers had hair total mercury levels in excess of 10 microg/g. There was a clear increase in hair mercury with reported fresh marine fish consumption."

"Mercury and DDT exposure risk to fish-eating human populations in Amazon." I. D. Rabitto, W. R. Bastos et al. *Environ Int.* 2010 Jul 26 (Epub ahead of print). Key finding: "Twenty-nine and thirty adults [of *Cichla monoculus* fish species] were collected respectively in February [rainy season] and August [dry season] 2007. A value of 48.2 percent and 33 percent of the individuals, respectively from rainy and dry seasons, presented mercury concentrations higher than the maximum established for safe human consumption. This fish species is an important vehicle for human exposure to mercury and DDTs."

"Neurobehavioral effects of prenatal exposure to methylmercury and PCBs and seafood intake: neonatal behavioral assessment scale results of Tohoku study of child development." K. Suzuki, K. Nakai, and T. Sugawara et al. *Environ Res.* 2010 Oct;110(7):699-704. Key finding: "We carried out a birth cohort study in a total of 498 mother-neonate pairs. The total mercury levels in maternal hair and in cord blood were analyzed. There was seen to be a positive association between maternal seafood intake and the motor cluster when considering the effects of mercury and PCBs. Our data suggest that prenatal exposure to methylmercury adversely affects neonatal neurobehavioral function. The neurobehavioral effect of prenatal exposure to PCBs remains unclear in our study."

"Mercury and polychlorinated biphenyls in Asian market fish: a response to results from mercury biomonitoring in New York City." W. McKelvey, M. Chang, J. Amason, N. Jeffery, J. Kricheff, and D. Kass. *Environ Res.* 2010 Oct;110(7):650-7. Key finding: "In 2004, the New York City Health and Nutrition Examination Survey measured the highest blood mercury levels in Asian and foreign-born Chinese demographic groups. Fish consumption was the strongest predictor of exposure. Our objective was to collect data on mercury contamination on fish species present in markets serving the Asian community. Mean mercury levels ranged from below the limit of detection in tilapia to the highest mercury level, which was measured in tilefish. Mean PCB levels ranged from 1 ng/g in red snapper to 98 ng/g in buffalo carp."

"Metal concentrations in monkfish (*Lophius americanus*) from the northeastern USA." A. K. Johnson, B. Bediako, and E. Wirth. *Environ Monit Assess.* 2010 Aug 18 (Epub ahead of print). Key finding: "Mercury levels were in excess of the maximum permissible limit for human consumption in American monkfish collected from Franklin Swell, Massachusetts; Mud Hole, New Jersey; and Fingers, Maryland, from February to May 2007."

"Blood total mercury and fish consumption in the Korean general population in KNHANES III, 2005." N. S. Kim and B. K. Lee. *Sci Total Environ.* 2010 Sep 15;408(20):4841–7. Key finding: "Among the nine listed individual types of fish and shellfish, there was a general trend for the blood mercury level to increase with the consumption frequency of squid, clam, salted seafood, and mackerel. The proportion of Korean women aged 20 to 49 years having blood mercury levels of at least 5.8 microg/L was 27.7 percent in our study."

"Prenatal and early childhood exposure to mercury and methylmercury in Spain, a high-fish-consumer country." S. Diez, S. Delgado et al. *Arch Environ Contam Toxicol.* 2009 Apr;56(3):615–22. Key finding: "Newborns from mothers who had intake of fish two or more times per week exhibited nearly threefold higher hair levels of total mercury than those who rarely or never consumed fish. Mercury levels in hair exceeded the EPA reference dose of 0.1 microg Hg/kg body weight per day in 42 percent of the population studied."

"Balancing the risks and the benefits of local fish consumption in Bermuda." E. Dewally, P. Touja et al. *Food Addit Contam Part A Chem Anal Control Expo Risk Assess.* 2008 Nov;25(11):1328–38. Key finding: "We have previously reported that some Bermudian neonates had elevated mercury in their umbilical blood compared with international guidelines. The objective of this study was to give precise and balanced information on the content of mercury, selenium, and PUFA in the most consumed fish species in Bermuda. Samples from 43 fish species were analyzed. Results show that mercury varies among species from 0.03 to 3.3 microg."

"Hair mercury levels in relation to fish consumption in a community of the Moroccan Mediterranean coast." H. Elhamri, L. Idrissi, M. Coquery et al. *Food Addit Contam.* 2007 Nov;24(11):1236–46. Key finding: "Based on fish consumption frequencies reported by 108 subjects included in the study, the weekly intake of methylmercury was estimated. Mercury concentrations in hair ranged from 0.22 to 9.56 microg g(-1) and were closely related to fish intake. Fishermen and their families consumed fish three to five times per week and were the most exposed population subgroup. A high proportion of women of child-bearing age (50 percent) had relatively high levels of mercury in their hair (3.08 to 7.88 microg g(-1)."

"Daily intake of arsenic, cadmium, mercury, and lead by consumption of edible marine species." G. Falco, J. M. Liobet, A. Bocio, and J. L. Domingo. *J Agric Food Chem.* 2006 Aug 9;54(16):6106–12. Key finding: "The estimated intake of methylmercury for boys in Catalonia, Spain, from consuming 14 edible marine species was 1.96 microg/kg/week, which was over the tolerable weekly intakes."

"Awareness of fish advisories and mercury exposure in women of childbearing age." S. Park and M. A. Johnson. *Nutr Rev.* 2006 May;64(5 Pt 1):250–6. Key finding: "Methylmercury crosses the placenta and increases the risk of impaired neurodevelopment in the fetus. Recent studies suggest that the awareness of fish advisories is low among women of childbearing age. Fish intake is strongly correlated with hair mercury concentrations. In women in states with fish advisories, hair mercury concentrations were 7-fold higher in women who consumed 20 or more servings of fish than in those who reported no fish consumption in the past 3 months. Among this high fish consumption group, hair mercury concentrations were up to 2.29 microg/g. This is of concern because the US EPA recommends that hair mercury be less than 1 microg/g."

"Fish intake, contaminants, and human health: evaluating the risks and the benefits." D. Mozaffarian and E. B. Rimm. *JAMA.* 2006 Oct 18;296(15):1885–99. Key finding: "We identified reports published through April 2006 evaluating (1) intake of fish or fish oil and cardiovascular risk (2) effects of methylmercury and fish oil on early neurodevelopment (3) risks of methylmercury for cardiovascular and neurologic outcomes in adults, and (4) health risks of dioxins and polychlorinated biphenyls in fish. Modest consumption of fish (e.g., 1 to 2 servings/wk), especially species higher in the n-3 fatty acids EPA and DHA, reduces risk of coronary death by 36 percent and total mortality by 17 percent and may favorably affect other clinical outcomes. Low-level methylmercury may adversely affect early neurodevelopment. Health effects of low-level methylmercury in adults are not clearly established. Methylmercury may modestly decrease the cardiovascular benefits of fish intake. Individuals with very high consumption should limit intake of species highest in mercury levels. Levels of dioxins and polychlorinated biphenyls in fish are low."

"Methylmercury exposure in Swedish women with high fish consumption." K. A. Bjornberg, M. Vahter, K. P. Grawe, and M. Berglund. *Sci Total Environ.* 2005 Apr 1;341(1–3):45–52. Key finding: "We studied the exposure to methylmercury in 127 Swedish women of childbearing age with average fish consumption of four times a week. Hair mercury levels exceeded the levels corresponding to the EPA reference dose of 0.1 microg MeHg/kg b.w. per day in 20 percent of the women. There seems to be no margin of safety for neurodevelopmental effects in fetus for women with high fish consumption unless they decrease their intake of certain fish species."

"Maternal and fetal mercury and n-3 polyunsaturated fatty acids as a risk and benefit of fish consumption to fetus." M. Sakamoto, M. Kubota, X. J. Liu, K. Murata, K. Nakai, and H. Satoh. *Environ Sci Technol.* 2004 Jul 15;38(14):3860–3. Key finding: "These results confirm that MeHg [methylmercury] which originated from fish consumption transferred from maternal to fetal circulation and existed in the fetal circulation with a positive correlation."

"Hair mercury levels in US children and women of childbearing age: reference range data from NHANES 1999–2000." M. A. McDowell, C. F. Dillon et al. *Environ Health Perspect.* 2004 Aug;112(11):1165–71. Key finding: "Exposure to methylmercury, a risk factor for neurodevelopmental toxicity, was assessed in 838 US children 1 to 5 years of age and in 1,726 women 16 to 49 years of age. Among frequent fish consumers, geometric mean hair mercury levels were 3-fold higher for women and 2-fold higher for children compared with nonconsumers."

"Blood mercury levels in US children and women of childbearing age, 1999–2000." S. E. Schober, T. H. Sinks, R. L. Jones, P. M. Bolger, M. McDowell, J. Osterloh, E. S. Garret, R. A. Canady, C. F. Dillon, Y. Sun, C. B. Joseph, and K. R. Mahaffey. *JAMA.* 2003 Apr 2;289(13):1667–74. Key finding: "Humans are exposed to methylmercury, a well-established neurotoxin, through fish consumption. The fetus is most sensitive to the adverse effects of exposure.1,250 children aged 1 to 5 years and 2,314 women aged 16 to 49 years were surveyed with household interviews, physical examinations, and blood mercury level assessments. Geometric mean mercury levels were almost 4-fold higher among women who ate 3 or more servings of fish in the past 30 days compared with women who ate no fish in that period. Approximately 8 percent of women had concentrations higher than the US Environmental Protection Agency's recommended reference dose (5.8 microg/L), below which exposures are considered without adverse effects."

"Organochlorine residues and elemental contaminants in US freshwater fish, 1976–1986; National Contaminant Biomonitoring Program." C. J. Schmitt, J. L. Zajicek, T. W. May, and D. F. Cowman. *Rev Environ Contam Toxicol.* 1999;162:43–104. Key finding: "The US Fish and Wildlife Service periodically determine concentrations of organochlorine chemical pesticide residues in freshwater fish collected from a nationwide network of stations. Concentrations of mercury and selenium were found to be high enough to constitute a threat."

Polycyclic Aromatic Hydrocarbon (PAH) Contamination of Fish

"Influence of smoking parameters on the concentration of polycyclic aromatic hydrocarbons (PAHs) in Danish smoked fish." L. Duedahl-Olesen et al. *Food Addit Contam Part A Chem Anal Control Expo Risk Assess.* 2010 Sep;27(9):1294–305. Key finding: "A new method for the analysis of 25 polycyclic aromatic hydrocarbon (PAH) compounds in fish was developed, validated, and used for the quantification of PAHs in 180 industrially smoked fish products. The sum concentration of 25 PAHs was highest in smoked herring and mackerel fillets with an average concentration of 320 and 235 microg/kg respectively. Increased combustion temperatures increased PAH levels."

"Determination of polycyclic aromatic hydrocarbons (PAHs) in commonly consumed Nigerian smoked/grilled fish and meat." V. O. Akpambang et al. *Food Addit Contam Part A Chem Anal Control Expo Risk Assess.* 2009 Jul;26(7):1096–103. Key finding: "Smoking and/or grilling, when carried out with traditional methods involving direct contact with wood combustion fumes, is responsible for high contamination levels with carcinogenic PAHs. The aim of this work was to investigate the PAH content of different smoked or grilled meat and fish products commonly consumed in Nigeria. Samples that were smoked or grilled using traditional methods were heavily contaminated with benzo(a)pyrene at levels ranging from 2.4 to 31.2 microg kg. This indicates a potential concern for consumer health."

"Polycyclic aromatic hydrocarbons in farmed rainbow trout (*Oncorhynchus mykiss*) processed by traditional flue gas smoking and by liquid smoke flavourings." P. Visciano, M. Perugini, F. Conte, and M. Amorena. *Food Chem Toxicol.* 2008 May;46(5):1409–13. Key finding: "Rainbow trout fillets processed by traditional gas smoking and by liquid smoke flavorings had PAH determined by high performance liquid chromatography. The following compounds were detected in all samples: anthracene, fluoranthene, pyrene, benz(a)anthracene, chrysene, benzo(b)fluoranthene, benzo(k)fluoranthene, and benzo(ghi)perylene. The results show that PAHs found in rainbow trout fillets could be considered as a consequence of environmental pollution and the mild smoking process described in the present study did not affect their concentrations."

"Polycyclic aromatic hydrocarbons in marine organisms from the Adriatic Sea, Italy." M. Perugini et al. *Chemosphere.* 2007 Jan;66(10):1904–10. Key finding: "Crustaceans and fish were analyzed and seven PAH compounds were detected in all samples. Atlantic mackerel, European hake, and blue whiting showed the highest PAH concentrations, ranging from 44.1 to 63.3 ngg(-1) wet weight."

"Polycyclic aromatic hydrocarbons in fresh and cold-smoked Atlantic salmon fillets." P. Visciano et al. *J Food Prot.* 2006 May;69(5):1134–8. Key finding: "The occurrence of PAHs in smoked fish as a consequence of cold smoking was studied. Raw fillets of *Salmo salar* from Norway or the Irish Sea were sampled in a modern smokehouse and examined for PAH content. A total of 11 PAH compounds were detected in both raw and smoked fillets. Results confirm that PAHs concentrations in smoked fish are the product of both sea pollution and the smoking process."

"Exposure to polycyclic aromatic hydrocarbons through consumption of edible marine species in Catalonia, Spain." J. M. Liobet, G. Falco, A. Bocio, and I. L. Domingo. *J Food Prot.* 2006 Oct;69(10):2493–9. Key finding: The concentrations of 16 PAH compounds were determined in samples of 14 edible marine species (sardine, tuna, anchovy, mackerel, swordfish, salmon, hake, red mullet, sole, cuttlefish, squid, clam, mussel, and shrimp). Mussel, clam, and shrimp had the highest PAH concentrations (22.4, 21.5, and 15.9 ng/g of fresh weight, respectively). The intake of benzo(a)pyrene and six other PAHs that are probably human carcinogens through consumption of these marine species would be associated with increase in the risk of development of cancer over a 70-year life span."

PCB, Dioxin, and Pesticide Contamination of Fish

"Perfluorinated compounds, polychlorinated biphenyls, and organochlorine pesticide contamination in composite food samples from Dallas, Texas, USA." A. Schecter, J. Colacino, D. Haffner, K. Patel, M. Opel, O. Papke, and L. Birnbaum. *Environ Health Perspect.* 2010 Jun;118(6):796–802. Key finding: "We measured concentrations of 32 organochlorine pesticides, 7 PCBs, and 11 PFCs in composite samples of 31 different types of food (310 individual food samples) purchased from supermarkets in Dallas. The highest level of pesticide contamination was from the DDT metabolite, which ranged from 0.028 ng/g weight in whole milk yogurt to 2.3 ng/g in catfish fillets. We found PCBs primarily in fish, with highest levels in salmon."

"Long-term effects of developmental exposure to low doses of PCB 126 and methylmercury." A. Vitalone, A. Catalani, C. Cinque, V. Fattori, P. Matteucci, A. R. Zuena, and L. G. Costa. *Toxicol Lett.* 2010 Aug 1;197(1):38–45. Key finding: "Methylmercury (MeHg) and polychlorinated biphenyls (PCBs) are food contaminants often found in fish. Experimental and epidemiological studies indicate that both are developmental neurotoxicants, and some reports suggest that they may cause additive and/or synergistic neurotoxicity. In this study behavioral alterations found in the first months of life in male rats exposed to PCB 126 or in female rats exposed to PCB 126 and methylmercury were persistent. Furthermore, an additional effect (increased body weight) was unmasked in adulthood in male rats exposed to PCB 126. These results indicate that developmental exposure to a low, environmentally relevant dose of PCB 126 causes long-lasting hyperactivity in male rats and a significant increase in body weight."

"Balancing the risk of dioxins and polychlorinated biphenyls (PCBs) and the benefit of long-chain polyunsaturated fatty acids of the n-3 variety for French fish consumers in western coastal areas." P. Verger, N. Khalfi, C. Roy et al. *Food Addit Contam Part A Chem Anal Control Expo Risk Assess.* 2008 Jun;25(6):765–71. Key finding: "A study of 401 fish-eating adults living in a coastal region of France was undertaken to establish exposure to dioxins/polychlorinated biphenyls and the intake of long-chain polyunsaturated fatty acids of the n-3 variety from fish consumption, which was estimated using food frequency diaries. Only 41 percent of these subjects had an optimal balance between the risk and benefit of eating fish, because 19 percent were meeting the nutritional recommendation but exceeding the toxicological threshold, whereas 38 percent were exposed below the toxicological threshold but failed to reach the recommended intake of long-chain n-3 polyunsaturated fatty acids. Similar results were found regarding the balance between long-chain n-3 polyunsaturated fatty acids and polychlorinated biphenyls even if a toxicological threshold was not established for these compounds."

"Consumption advisories for salmon based on risk of cancer and noncancer health effects." X. Huang, R. A. Hites et al. *Environ Res.* 2006 Jun;101(2):263–74. Key finding: "The levels of dioxins, furans, PCBs, and chlorinated pesticides were determined in farmed salmon for eights regions in Europe, North America, and South America, in salmon fillets purchased in 16 cities in Europe and North America, and in five species of wild Pacific salmon. Upon application of US Environmental Protection Agency methods for developing fish consumption advisories for cancer from mixtures of all of these substances for which US

EPA has reported a cancer slope factor, the most stringent recommendation for farmed salmon from northern Europe was for consumption of at most one meal every 5 months in order to not exceed an elevated risk of cancer of more than 1 in 100,000. Farmed salmon from North and South America triggered advisories of between 0.4 and one meal per month. Retail market samples in general reflected levels found in regionally farmed fish, although much of the US salmon comes from Chile, which had somewhat lower contaminant levels than the North American farmed samples. Even wild salmon triggered advisories of between one and less than five meals per month."

"Exposure to polychlorinated biphenyls (PCBs) in food and cancer risk: recent advances." A. M. Roveda, L. Veronesi, R. Zoni, M. E. Colucci, and G. Sansebastiano. *Sanita Pubbl.* (Italian) 2006 Nov-Dec;62(6):677–96. Key finding: "Humans continue to be exposed to the toxic effects of PCBs because of their resistance to chemical and biological decomposition, their capacity of bioaccumulation, and their long half-life. Studies performed so far have pointed out a possible association between exposure to PCBs and increased risk of developing breast, prostate, testicular, ovarian, and uterine cancers. These compounds may also act as [endocrine disruptors] and cause infertility. PCBs accumulate in organisms through the food chain, and food accounts for 90 percent of exposure. The highest concentrations being found in fish (such as salmon and shellfish), dairy products (especially milk and butter), and animal fat."

"Fish intake, contaminants, and human health: evaluating the risks and the benefits." D. Mozaffarian and E. B. Rimm. *JAMA.* 2006 Oct 18;296(15):1885–99. Key finding: "We identified reports published through April 2006 evaluating (1) intake of fish or fish oil and cardiovascular risk (2) effects of methylmercury and fish oil on early neurodevelopment (3) risks of methylmercury for cardiovascular and neurologic outcomes in adults, and (4) health risks of dioxins and polychlorinated biphenyls in fish. Modest consumption of fish (e.g., 1 to 2 servings/wk), especially species higher in the n-3 fatty acids EPA and DHA, reduces risk of coronary death by 36 percent and total mortality by 17 percent and may favorably affect other clinical outcomes. Low-level methylmercury may adversely affect early neurodevelopment. Health effects of low-level methylmercury in adults are not clearly established. Methylmercury may modestly decrease the cardiovascular benefits of fish intake. Individuals with very high consumption should limit intake of species highest in mercury levels. Levels of dioxins and polychlorinated biphenyls in fish are low."

"Fish intake and serum levels of organochlorines among Japanese women." H. Tsukino, T. Hanaoka, H. Sasaki et al. *Sci Total Environ.* 2006 Apr 15;359(1-3):90–100. Key finding: "This study evaluates background serum levels of selected organochlorine compounds among Japanese women of reproductive age. A cross-sectional study was performed on 80 Japanese women, aged 26 to 43 years, who complained of infertility and were confirmed to have endometriosis. The serum levels of total toxic equivalency of PCDDs, PCDFs, PCBs, and 13 chlorinated pesticides or their metabolites were measured. The present study suggests that Japanese women who consume fish frequently in their reproductive period tend to accumulate organochlorines in their bodies."

"Persistent organic pollutants and heavy metals in typical seafoods consumed in Singapore." S. Bayen, E. Koroleva, H. K. Lee, and J. P. Obbard. *J Toxicol Environ Health A.* 2005 Feb 13;68(3):151–66. Key finding: "In this study, the levels of several heavy metals and persistent organic pollutants were measured in the edible portions of 20 different seafood types consumed in Singapore. Daily intake of DDTs, heptachlor, and PCBs in seafood exceeded the conservative cancer benchmark concentrations set by the US Environmental Protection Agency, suggesting that a significant number of people are potentially at risk in Singapore over a lifetime from seafood consumption."

"Human exposure to dioxins through the diet in Catalonia, Spain: carcinogenic and non-carcinogenic risk." J. M. Llobet, J. L. Domingo, A. Bocio, C. Casas, A. Teixido, and L. Muller. *Chemosphere.* 2003 Mar;50(9):1193–200. Key finding: "Food samples were randomly acquired in seven cities of Catalonia. Dioxin concentrations were determined in 108 samples belonging to the following groups: vegetables, fruits, pulses, cereals, fish and shellfish, meats and meat products, eggs, milk and dairy products, and oil and fats. Fish and shellfish had the highest concentrations in total dietary intake (31 percent) with dairy products (25 percent) and cereals (14 percent) and meat (13 percent) showing the greatest percentages of contribution to dioxin intake. The carcinogenic risk level was 1,360 excess cancer over a lifetime of 70 years."

"Fish intake, plasma omega-3 polyunsaturated fatty acids, and polychlorinated dibenzo-p-dioxins/polychlorinated dibenzo-furans and co-planar polychlorinated biphenyls in the blood of the Japanese population." K. Arisawa, T. Matsumura, C. Tohyama, H. Saito, H. Satoh, M. Nagai, M. Morita, and T. Suzuki. *Int Arch Occup Environ Health.* 2003 Apr;76(3):205–15. Key finding: "A cross-sectional study was performed on 131 men and 122 women (aged 20 to 76 years) who resided in five prefectures of Japan and had no occupational exposure to dioxins. The frequency of intake of coastal fish such as horse mackerel and sardine was associated with concentrations of polychlorinated dioxins. The level of intake of marine fish, especially raw fish and coastal varieties, may be associated with increased blood levels of dioxin-related compounds. Despite high fish consumption in Japan, the body burden of dioxins in the population was not found to be higher than that in western countries."

"Impairments of memory and learning in older adults exposed to polychlorinated biphenyls via consumption of Great Lakes fish." S. L. Schantz and D. M. Gasior et al. *Environmental Health Perspectives.* 2001 Jun;109(5):605. Key finding: "An association between in utero PCB exposure and impaired childhood intellectual functioning has been reported, but the potential impact of PCB exposure during adulthood on intellectual functioning has received little attention. We assessed the impact of PCBs and other fish-borne contaminants on intellectual functioning in older adults. The subjects were 49- to 86-year-old Michigan residents. Fish eaters ate >24 lb of sport-caught Lake Michigan fish per year and non-fish eaters ate six pounds of fish per year. A battery of cognitive tests including tests of memory and learning, executive function, and visual-spatial function was administered to 180 subjects (101 fish eaters and 79 non-fish eaters.) Blood samples were analyzed for PCBs and 10 other contaminants. PCNS and DDE were markedly elevated in fish eaters. After controlling for potential confounders PCB, but not DDE, exposure was associated with lower scores on several measures of memory and learning. In conclusion, PCB exposure during adulthood was associated with impairments in memory and learning. These results are consistent with previous research showing an association between in utero PCB exposure and impairments of memory during infancy and childhood."

Toxic Metals Contamination of Seafood

"Analysis of toxic metals in seafood sold in New York State by inductively coupled plasma mass spectrometry and direct combustion analysis." T. J. King, R. S. Sheridan, and D. H. Rice. *J Food Prot.* 2010 Sep;73(9):1715–20. Key finding: "Concentrations of 12 metals (As, Be, Cd, Cr, Pb, Mo, Ni, Tl, Th, U, V, Hg) were determined in samples of fish and lobster obtained from various stores and markets in New York State. A total of 177 fish and lobster samples were initially analyzed. Twenty-two samples had mercury concentrations greater than the 1,000 ng/g limit set by the Commission of the European Communities. The highest Cd concentration (511 ng/g) was found in lobster; this level is greater than the 500 ng/g limit set by the Commission of the European Communities. The highest average mercury level (1,190 ng/g) was found in swordfish. The highest arsenic level (13,400 ng/g) was found in monkfish."

"Heavy metals in Pacific cod (*Gadus macrocephalus*) from the Aleutians: location, age, size, and risk." J. Burger, M. Gochfeld, T. Shukla et al. *J Toxicol Environ Health A.* 2007 Nov;70(22):1897–911. Key finding: "If a subsistence fisher from one of the Aleut villages ate one meal (8 ounces) of cod per week, they would exceed the US EPA reference adverse dose for arsenic and mercury."

"Daily intake of arsenic, cadmium, mercury, and lead by consumption of edible marine species." G. Falco, J. M. Liobet, A. Bocio, and J. L. Domingo. *J Agric Food Chem.* 2006 Aug 9;54(16):6106–12. Key finding: "The estimated intake of methylmercury for boys in Catalonia, Spain, from consuming 14 edible marine species was 1.96 microg/kg/week, which was over the tolerable weekly intakes."

"Organochlorine residues and elemental contaminants in US freshwater fish, 1976-1986; National Contaminant Biomonitoring Program." C. J. Schmitt, J. L. Zajicek, T. W. May, and D. F. Cowman. *Rev Environ Contam Toxicol.* 1999;162:43–104. Key finding: "The US Fish and Wildlife Service periodically determine concentrations of organochlorine chemical pesticide residues in freshwater fish collected from a nationwide network of stations. Concentrations of mercury and selenium were found to be high enough to constitute a threat."

PFO Contamination of Fish and Hypolipidemia

"Effects of perfluorooctanesulfonate exposure on plasma lipid levels in the Inuit population of Nunavik (Northern Quebec)." M. L. Chateau-Degat, D. Pereg, R. Dallaire, P. Ayotte, S. Dery, and E. Dewailly. *Environ Res.* 2010 Aug 7(Epub ahead of print). Key finding: "Perfluorooctanesulfonate (PFOS) is used as a surfactant in various commercial products. In rodents, exposure to this compound induced various health effects, including hypolipidemia. A recent study reported an increase in plasma cholesterol associated with exposure to perfluorinated compounds in humans exposed through drinking water. The Inuit of Nunavik are exposed to environmental contaminants through the consumption of fish and game. Plasma concentrations of PFOS and lipids were assessed in Nunavik Inuit adults in the framework of a large-scale environmental health study. The results of this study show a relationship between PFOS and plasma lipid levels."

Glossary

Aldrin. Aldrin is an insecticide.

Alkylphenols. A family of surfactants, alkylphenols are ingredients in detergents and other consumer products.

Alpha-linolenic acid (ALA). ALA is a type of omega-3 fatty acid that is found in plants, especially marine algae. ALA provides the human body with the other two types of omega-3s (DHA and EPA).

Anisakid nematodes. One family of worms that can infect salmon, sardines, squid, and cuttlefish (and the people who eat them) is classified as anisakid nematodes.

Aquaculture: Aquaculture means aquafarming or fish farming.

Aquafarming: Aquafarming means aquaculture or fish farming.

Beta-methylamino-L-alanine (BMAA). An environmental toxin produced by cyanobacteria is called BMAA.

Bioaccumulation. When a substance accumulates in body tissue at a higher concentration than in the surrounding environment, the process is called bioaccumulation.

Biomagnification. The ability of pollutants to become more concentrated as they are absorbed up the food chain is known as biomagnification.

Bisphenol A. Also known as BPA, bisphenol A is a chemical compound used to make polycarbonate plastic. It is found in the lining of food cans.

Body burden. The term body burden refers to a buildup of heavy metals and synthetic chemicals in human or animal bodies.

Carcinogen. A substance that causes cancer is called a carcinogen.

Ciguatera poisoning. Caused by ciguatoxin, ciguatera food poisoning occurs when people eat contaminated reef fish.

Cyanobacteria. Also called blue-green algae, cyanobacteria is a photosynthetic bacteria eaten by sea life.

DDD. Short for dichlorodiphenyldichloroethane, DDD is a metabolite of DDT.

DDE. Short for dichlorodiphenyldichloroethylene, DDE is a metabolite of DDT.

DDT. Short for dichlorodiphenyltrichloroethane, DDT is an insecticide.

Dieldrin. Dieldrin is an insecticide.

Dinoflagellates. A form of plankton that is eaten by fish, dinoflagellates carry ciguatoxin, which causes ciguatera poisoning (see page 145).

Dioxins. Dioxins are toxic by-products of industrial processes, including waste incineration and chlorine bleaching of paper and textiles.

Diphyllobothrium. A type of tapeworm that is found in certain fish, such as salmon, trout, and perch, and can infect humans is called diphyllobothrium.

Docosahexaenoic acid (DHA). DHA is a type of omega-3 fatty acid.

EE2. Otherwise known as 17alpha-ethinylestradiol, EE2 is a synthetic estrogen used in contraceptives.

Eicosapentaenoic acid (EPA). EPA is a type of omega-3 fatty acid.

Fauna: Fauna is animal life.

Food chain. The food chain is an order of predation in which "higher" life forms use "lower" members as food sources.

Frankenfish. Reminiscent of Frankenstein's monster, "Frankenfish" is a term used to refer to fish that are genetically modified or contaminated with industrial toxins, including heavy metals and chemicals.

Intersex. An intersex individual displays characteristics of both genders, such as a male fish who carries eggs.

Mirex. Mirex is an insecticide.

Mutagenic. An agent that increases the frequency or extent of mutation is mutagenic.

Organochlorines. Chlorinated hydrocarbons that are typically used as pesticides (such as aldrin, DDT, and dieldrin) are categorized as organochlorines.

Oxybenzone. A chemical found in sunscreens, oxybenzone is a documented hormone disrupter.

Perfluorinated compounds (PFCs). PFCs are water- and stain-repellent chemicals.

Persistent organic pollutants (POPs). POPs are toxic compounds that do not degrade in the environment.

Phthalates. Phthalates are used widely as plasticizers and as solvents in products such as perfumes and cosmetics.

Polybrominated diphenyl ethers (PBDEs). PBDEs are flame retardants.

Polychlorinated biphenyls (PCBs). PCBs are compounds that have various industrial applications, especially as coolants.

Polycyclic aromatic hydrocarbons (PAHs). PAHs are by-products of burning fuels.

Scombroid poisoning. Caused by scombrotoxin, scombroid poisoning typically occurs when people consume fish that has been inadequately refrigerated and allowed to spoil.

Toxaphene. Toxaphene is an insecticide.

Transgenic. A being is defined as transgenic when genes from another organism have been incorporated into it.

Triclosan. An antifungal and antibacterial agent, triclosan is used in dozens of consumer products, such as mouthwash, shaving cream, toothpaste, and deodorant.

Wasabi. A condiment made from a plant root, wasabi kills microbes and is commonly served with sushi to reduce the risk of food poisoning.

Index

mercury in, 80–81
PBDEs in, 82
PCBs in, 78
pesticides in, 82, 83, 84
rainbow trout, PAHs in, 136–37
salmon
 aldrin in, 84
 cancer risk and, 82, 83
 dangers of, 77–79
 dieldrin in, 82, 84
 dioxins in
  Carpenter, David O., and, 78
  as common, 84
  Environmental Health Perspectives
   and, 82
  Environmental Research and, 26, 138
 furans in, 138
 genetically engineered (GE) fish and, 91
 mirex in, 84
 overfishing and, 88, 89
 PBDEs in, 36, 84
 PCBs in
  cancer and, 138
  as common, 84
  distribution chain and, 78
  fish skin and, 36
  research about, 81
  vs. wild salmon, 82
 pesticides in, 138
 as tainted, 77
 toxaphene in, 78, 82, 84
 wild-caught vs., 80
 shrimp, overfishing and, 88
 tilapia, 80
 toxaphene in, 78
 wild-caught fish vs., 77, 108
fat (dietary), 26, 109, 129
fat cells, chemical accumulation in, 4
fatigue, from parasite, 38
fauna (animals), 91, 98, 100, 146
FDA (US Food and Drug Administration)
 BPA and, 51
 fish consumption advisories and, 79
 genetically engineered fish and, 90, 92
 mercury and
  bluefin akami, 34, 35
  contamination guidelines, 6, 7
  in tuna, 20
 Office of Biotechnology, 91
 PCBs and, 82
 salmon consumption and, vi
 sushi and, 32, 33
Fenton, Jennifer, 62
fertility issues, 35, 130, 139, 140
fibrocystic disease, fish consumption and, 130
fibromyalgia, marine algae/sea vegetables for, 109
finfish, 18, 88
Fingers (MD), mercury in monkfish and, 133
Finland, studies in, 22, 59
Fish and Fisheries, vii
Fish and Wildlife Conservation Commission, 12

fish ear bones, harm to, 101
fisheries
 aquaculture's effect on, 88, 89
 Atlantic salmon and, 91
 decline in fish population and, 87, 96
 Fisheries and Oceans Canada, 91
 recommendations for, 104
 World Review of Fisheries and Aquaculture, 89
fish farming. *See* aquaculture (aqua farming/fish
  farming)
fish-free diet, 109
fish meal, 79, 88, 89, 108
fish migratory patterns, 102
fish oil/fish oil supplements
 about, 61–62
 Alzheimer's disease and, 64–65
 artery inflammation and, 66
 athletic performance and, 63
 cancer and, 62–63, 65
 EPA (eicosapentaenoic acid) in, 146
 farm-raised fish and, 108
 heart (cardiovascular/coronary) disease and,
  66–68, 134, 139
 immune system and, 65
 overfishing and, 88, 89
 plants vs., 68
 pregnancy and, 64
Fitzgerald, Randall *(The Hundred Year Lie),* 49
flame retardants
 in farm-raised fish, 82
 as health threat, 26–27, 28
 in Oregon rivers, 45
 PBDEs, 147
 sushi and, 35
 as travelers, 1, 3
flatfish, endocrine disruptors in, 47
flaxseeds/flaxseed oil, as fish oil supplement
  alternative, 61–62, 70
fliers, 1, 2, 3
Florida, BP oil spill contaminants and, 14
Florida Department of Health fish advisories,
  12–13
fluoxetine, as endocrine disruptor, 55
Foer, Jonathan Safran *(Eating Animals),* vii
follicular cancer, fish consumption and, 130
Food Additives & Contaminants, 133, 136, 138
Food and Agricultural Organization (FAO), 34
food chain, 108, 139, 146
Food IS Medicine: The Scientific Evidence
  (Clement), 72, 109
food poisoning, 17–19, 37, 147
forage fish, 79, 89
France
 contaminated salmon in, 78
 dioxin study and, 138
 fish oil supplement study and, 63
 PCB study and, 138
 sarpa salpa hallucinogenic poisoning in, 102
 sushi diphyllobothrium in, 38
Frankenfish, 32, 90–92, 146
Frankfurt (Germany), contaminated salmon in, 78

Franklin Swell (MA), mercury in monkfish and, 133
freshwater fish
contraceptive EE2 in, 52
mercury/methylmercury in, 4, 5, 136, 142
pesticides in, 136, 142
selenium in, 142
fungicides, 1, 3
furans, in salmon, 25, 138

G

gar, Florida fish advisory about, 12
gas & oil exploration, oceans' health and, 100, 104
gastric cancer, fish consumption and, 130
GE (genetically engineered) fish, 90–92
"gender-bender" fish, 13
genetic abnormalities/alterations, to fish, 14, 107
genetically engineered (GE) fish, 90–92
genetically modified animals/crops/plants, 80, 90, 91, 146
genetic diversity, loss of, 97
genital deformities, endocrine disruptors and, 42
Germany, 36, 37, 78, 99
global outcomes, oceans' health and, 97
global warming, 9, 101
GloFish, 91
Gochfeld, Michael, 33, 34
gold mining, mercury contamination and, 6
Gore-Tex, 3
government subsidies, for fishing, 103–4
gray prawns, 10
Great Lakes
carp and, 103
mercury contamination in, 5–6
PCBs and, 25, 141
toxaphene in, 8
Greenland ice sheet melting, 97
green mussels, 10
grilled fish, PAHs and, 136
Grossman, Elizabeth *(Chasing Molecules)*, 1
grouper, mercury in, 7
Guadiana River (Portugal), endocrine disruptors in, 49
Guardian (London), 101

H

hair spray chemicals, as endocrine disruptors, 50
hake, PAHs in, 137
halibut, 7, 131
hallucinations/hallucinogenic poison, 18, 102
Hamilton Harbour (Canada), SSRIs in, 55
Harvard Medical School, 77–78
Harvard School of Public Health, 67
HCB (hexachlorobenzene), 3, 9, 11, 83
HCH (hexachlorocyclohexane), 3, 11
Health, 19
Health Canada, 34
Health Department fish advisories, 12

heart (cardiovascular/coronary artery) disease
bioaccumulation and, 36
canned tuna as risk for, 33
DHA and, 139
EPA (eicosapentaenoic acid) and, 139
farm-raised fish and, 81
fish oil and, 66–68, 134, 139
mercury consumption and
high intake and, 22, 34, 35
increased risk and, 131
JAMA report about, 134
methylmercury and, 139
omega-3 fatty acids and, 57, 58, 59, 131
overconsumption of fish and, vi
PCBs and, 24, 25
physician recommendations about eating fish and, 19–20
tilapia and, 60–61
vegetarianism and, 109
walnuts to reduce risk of, 74
heart rate problems, from parasites, 38
hempseeds, as fish oil supplement alternative, 62
heptachlor, 3, 10, 140
herbicides, 1, 3, 99
herbs, for bacteria/parasite cleansing, 39
herring/smoked herring, 11, 58, 89
hexachlorobenzene (HCB), as traveler, 3
hexachlorocyclohexane (HCH), as traveler, 3
Hg (mercury). *See* mercury (Hg)
high blood pressure, 72, 109
high cholesterol, marine algae/sea vegetables for, 109
Holland, anisakid nematode poisoning in, 38
hoppers, 1, 2, 3, 14
hormone-disrupting chemicals, vi, 44, 45
horse mackerel, contaminants in, 10, 140
human activities/human-caused disruptions, 96–97, 100–102
Hundred Year Lie, The (Fitzgerald), 49
Hunters Lake (FL), fish advisories for, 12
Huron, Lake, organochlorines in, 8
Hurricane Floyd, 101
hyperactivity, PBDEs/PCBs and, 27, 138
hypoxia (oxygen loss), oceans' health and, 97

I

IBC Library Series, 72–73
immune system/immune system disorders
bioaccumulation and, 36
BP oil spill and, 14
dioxins and, 26
farm-raised salmon and, 79
fish oil and, 65
marine algae and, 72–73
organic pollutants and, 2
from parasite, 38
PCBs and, 24
sushi consumption and, 35
industrial chemicals/pollutants. *See also* specific types of
about, 99

in farm-raised fish, 81
fliers, swimmers, and hoppers in, 1, 2
Frankenfish and, 146
increase in, vi, 35
in sushi, 32
Industrial Revolution, 101
infectious salmon anemia, 84
infertility, 130, 139, 140
inflammation of the arteries, fish oil and, 66
insecticides, 53–54, 145, 146. *See also* specific
types of
Institute for Food Quality and Food Safety, 36
Institute for Health and the Environment, 78
Institute of Environmental Medicine, 21
Institute of Human Nutrition, 63
insulin levels, 68, 74
*International Archives of Occupational and
Environmental Health,* 140–41
International Journal of Food Microbiology, 18,
31, 38
*International Journal of Hygiene and
Environmental Health,* 81
International Programme on the State of the
Ocean, 95, 104
International Society for the Study of Fatty Acids
and Lipids conference, 63, 65
International Union for Conservation of Nature,
95
intersex fish/organs
alkylphenol/phthalates and, 46–47, 51
BPA and, 47, 51–52
contraceptive EE2 and, 52
defined, 146
endocrine disruptors and, 45, 46, 48–49, 50
genetically engineered (GE) fish and, 92
insecticides/pesticides and, 54
PCBs and, 53
pharmaceutical/prescription drugs and, 42, 44
in South Africa, 47
Inuit, PFOS (perfluorooctanesulfonate) and, 142
invasive species, deep seas and, 98
IQ problems, 11, 27
Iranian pregnancy/mercury consumption study,
132
Ireland, endocrine disruptors in, 46–47
Irish Sea, 47, 137
irritable bowel syndrome, marine algae/sea
vegetables for, 109
irritableness, from parasites, 38
Israel, jellyfish in, 101
Italian PAH studies, 23, 137
Italy, endocrine disruptors in, 47

J

*JAMA (Journal of the American Medical
Association)*
fish contamination/human health report/
study in, 134, 139
fish oil/Alzheimer's disease study in, 64
mercury finding reported in, 135
SSRIs' study in, 54

Japan/Japanese
anisakid nematode poisoning in, 38
coastal study, 10
dioxins and, 140–41
earthquake/tsunami, radioactivity and, 14
fish oil study findings and, 63, 65
mercury and, 21, 34
pesticide study and, 140
sushi, 32
Java Sea, overfishing in, 87
jellyfish population, 101
Jourdois, Benedicte, 33
Journal of Agricultural and Food Chemistry,
26–27, 134, 142
Journal of Food Protection, 137
Journal of Medicinal Food, 72
Journal of Neuroscience, 73
Journal of the American Dietetic Association, 60
*Journal of the American Medical Association
(JAMA). See* JAMA (*Journal of the American
Medical Association*)
Journal of Toxicology and Environmental Health,
27, 142

K

kale, as omega-3 fatty acid source, 71
Kidd, Karen, 48
king mackerel, mercury in, 7
Knuth, Barbara, 79
Korean fish consumption/contamination, 133
krill/krill oil, 13, 70, 79
Kristof, Nicholas D., 42

L

labeling of fish, 77, 92
lake fish, PCBs in, 8
lake trout, 8, 9
land/river catchment management, 104
largemouth bass, 11, 12, 28, 53
Las, Vegas (NV), canned tuna/mercury study
in, 131
Latin America, sushi diphyllobothrium in, 38
learning impairment, PCBs and, 24–25
leukemia study, smoked fish and, 129
Lexapro, as endocrine disruptor, 54
LifeGive Par-A-Gon, 39
Linus Pauling Institute, 58, 70
Lipids, 65
Listeria monocytogenes, 36, 37
listeriosis, 37
litter and waste, in deep seas, 98
liver disease, 14, 24
lobster/lobster die-off, 100, 141
Long Island Sound, lobster die-off in, 100–101
Los Angeles County (CA) wastewater falls,
endocrine disruptors in, 50
lost ships, pollution decay from, 99
Lou Gehrig's disease, seafood and, 27
Louisiana, BP oil spill contaminants and, 14
lung disease, BP oil spill and, 14

Luvuhu River (South Africa), endocrine disruptors in, 47

M

mackerel. *See also* specific types of
  jellyfish vs., in Cardigan Bay (Wales), 101
  mercury in, 133
  PAHs in, 23, 137
  PCBs/PCDFs in, 10
  scromboid food poisoning and, 19
Mahaffey, Kate, 22
mahi mahi, scromboid food poisoning and, 19
Maine, 36, 81
marine algae
  about, 70–73
  ALA in, 145
  as alternative to eating fish, 108
  food chain and, 58
  health benefits of, 109
  as omega-3 fatty acid source, 59, 89, 108
marine environment, protecting, 104
Marine Environmental Research Institute, 36
Marine Pollution Bulletin, 131
Maryland, contaminated monkfish in, 133
Massachusetts, contaminated fish in, 78, 133
meat consumption/meat-eating diet
  cancer and, 109, 129, 130
  diabetes and, 109
  dioxins and, 140
  heart disease and, 109
  high blood pressure and, 109
  leukemia risk and, 129
  vegetarian diet vs., 109, 110
medaka fish, 46
Mediterranean fish, 87, 99, 102, 133–34
MeHg (methylmercury). *See* methylmercury (MeHg)
memory impairment, PCBs and, 24–25
mental retardation, mercury and, 35
mercury (Hg). *See also* in specific types of fish
  in Amazon, 132
  biomagnification and, 13–14
  in Canadian Arctic/subarctic regions, 9
  cooking's effect on, 23
  in Donner Lake (CA), 9
  in fish oil supplements, 61
  gold mining and, 6
  as health threat, 19–23
  increase in emissions of, 5
  levels, 7
  omega-3 fatty acids and, 22
  pregnancy and
    in California, 6
    findings/reports about
      Archives of Environmental Contamination & Toxicology, 133
      Environmental Health Perspectives, 135
      Environmental Science & Technology, 135

warning labels about, lack of, vi
  "safe" consumption of, 6–7
  study about, 5
  Taiwanese study about, 20–21, 131
  testing, lack of, 22
  as toxic, vi, 1
  as traveler, 3
  in United States, 5–6
metal(s)
  body burden and, 43, 145
  Frankenfish and, 146
  in monkfish, 133
  poisoning from, 19
  in Singaporean seafood study, 10
  in sushi, 32
  as waste, in deep seas, 98, 99
methane, from sea beds, 97
methylmercury (MeHg)
  in Catalonia (Spain), 134
  as common contaminant, 36
  in freshwater fish, 5
  heart (cardiovascular/coronary artery) disease and, 139
  mercury and, 4
  in Moroccan coastal community, 133–34
  neurological problems and, 139
  as neurotoxicant, 138
  pregnancy and
    fish advisories and, 134
    JAMA reports/studies about, 134, 135, 139
    neurobehavioral function and, 132
    Spanish study, 133
    Swedish study, 135
    transference and, 21
  Spanish study about, 142
  as traveler, 3
Mexico, Gulf of, 14, 89–90, 99, 100
Mexico City (Mexico), gastric cancer study in, 130
Michigan, Lake, 8, 25, 141
Michigan PCB study, 24–25
Michigan State University, 62
migration, of carp, 102–3
Mila (company), 70
Miller, Henry I., 91
mining waste/deep-sea mining, 98, 100
minnows, endocrine disruptors in, 48
mirex
  in Aleutian Island waters (AK), 9
  bioaccumulation of, 54
  defined, 146
  in farm-raised fish, 83, 84
Mississippi River, carp as invasive species in, 102
Mississippi State Chemical Laboratory, 52
Mobile River Basin (AL), PCBs in, 53
Mohawk Indian disease/PCBs' study, 25
Monbiot, George, 101
monkfish, arsenic/mercury in, 133, 142
Montreal (Canada), studies in, 43, 130
moray eel, ciguatera poisoning and, 18
Morocco, mercury in fish and, 133–34

Mud Hole (NJ), mercury in monkfish and, 133
multiple sclerosis misdiagnosis, ciguatera
   poisoning and, 18
muscle aches, ciguatera poisoning and, 18
muscle weakness, from parasites, 38
mussels, 11, 28, 137
mustard oil, as omega-3 fatty acid source, 70
mutagenic, 23, 147

N

National Breast Screening Study, 130
National Contaminant Biomonitoring Program,
   136
National Geographic, 13, 87
National Geographic News, 48, 100
National Institute on Aging, 64
National Marine Fishery Service, 103
National Oceanic and Atmospheric
   Administration (NOAA), 80
Native American diabetes'/PCBs' study, 25
Nature, 79, 88, 89, 91
nausea, 18, 38
negative synergies, human diet and, 107
nervous system disorders, bioaccumulation
   and, 36
neurological development/disorders/problems
   ciguatera poisoning and, 18
   farm-raised salmon and, 79
   mercury consumption and
      Biology Letters report about, 34
      EPA (US Environmental Protection
         Agency) and, 21
      JAMA report about, 134
      Marine Pollution Bulletin report about,
         131
      tuna sushi and, 35
   methylmercury and, 138, 139
   omega-3 fatty acids and, 58
   overconsumption of fish and, vi
   PCBs and
      as common, 11, 53
      fat tissues and, 24
      Michigan, Lake, study and, 141
      Toxicology Letters report about, 138
   spinach and, 73
Nevada, canned tuna/mercury study in, 131
New England, 87, 90
New Jersey, 34, 133
New York/New York City
   food poisoning outbreaks in, 18
   mercury testing in, 34
   metals in fish samples in, 141–42
   New York City Health and Nutrition
      Examination Survey, 132
   sushi testing in, 32–33
New York Times articles
   endocrine disruptors, 42
   lobster die-off, 100–101
   mercury, 22
   sushi, 32, 33

Nigerian smoked fish, PAHs and, 136
NOAA (National Oceanic and Atmospheric
   Administration), 80
Nobel Prize, 53
norfluoxetine, as endocrine disruptor, 55
North America
   consumption of fish in, v
   contaminated salmon distributed from, 78
   diphyllobothrium in, 38
   salmon studies in, 25, 138, 139
North Pacific Ocean, genetically engineered (GE)
   fish in, 91
North Sea (Europe), 47, 87
Norway, 78, 81, 84, 137
numbness, 18, 38
Nunavik Inuit, PFOS and, 142
Nutrition, 72
Nutrition and Cancer, 74
Nutrition Review, 134

O

obesity, marine algae/sea vegetables for, 109
ocean (saltwater) fish/ocean-caught fish, 4,
   35–36, 90
oceans' health. *See also* overfishing
   about, 95–96
   acidification, 101
   climate change and, 96
   deep seas
      Census of Marine Life and, 97
      deep-sea mining and, 100
      dredge in, 98
      industrial chemicals in, 99, 100
      litter and waste in, 98
      lost ship pollution decay in, 100
      mining waste in, 98
      oil & gas exploration and, 100
      pharmaceuticals in, 98–99
      radioactive waste in, 99
      sewage in, 98
   global outcomes and, 97
   human activities and, 96–97, 100–102
   hypoxia and, 97
   invasive species and, 102–3
   scientists' recommendations about, 104
   tax subsidies and, 103–4
octyl-methoxycinnamate, as endocrine disruptor,
   49–50
oil & gas exploration, oceans' health and, 100,
   104
Ojibwa tribe, 8
omega-3 fatty acids. *See also* specific types of
   cancer and, 65
   fish oil supplements and, 61–62
   government agencies and, vi
   as "healthy," 57–59
   heart (cardiovascular/coronary) disease and,
      66–68
   mercury negating benefit of, 22
   PEOs and, 68–69

Reviews on Environmental Health, 24, 35–36
rheumatoid arthritis, omega-3 fatty acids and, 58
river/land catchment management, 104
Robert Wood Johnson Medical School, 33
rock sole, PCBs in, 10
rolled sushi, 31
Romanian Danube Delta, contaminants found in, 10–11
Rowen, Robert, 68–69
Royal Victoria Hospital (Canada), 72–73

S

Sacramento-San Joaquin River Delta (CA), mercury in, 6
safety of eating fish, 107–8
salmon. *See also* specific types of
  anisakid nematodes and, 145
  aquaculture of, 77–80
  cancer risk and, 25
  chlordane in, 10
  consumption increase in, v
  DDT in, 10
  dioxins in, 25, 26
  diphyllobothrium in, 38, 146
  endocrine disruptors in, 45
  "fresh," 77
  furans in, 25, 138
  government subsidies and, 103–4
  heavy metals in, 10
  mercury in, 131
  omega-3 fatty acid and, v, 58, 131
  overconsumption, vi
  PAHs in, 23, 137
  parasites in, 38
  PBDEs in, 36
  PCBs in
    cancer and, 130, 139
    in Dallas (TX), 137
    FDA/USDA and, vi
    Singaporean study about, 10
    wild salmon vs. farm-raised salmon, 36
  pesticides in, 25
  pollutants in, vi
  POPs in, 10
  sushi/sushi rolls, 31, 35
  toxaphene and, 8
salmonella, 36, 37
salted seafood, mercury in, 133
saltwater (ocean) fish/ocean-caught fish, 4, 35–36, 90
San Diego (CA) wastewater falls, endocrine disruptors in, 50
San Francisco (CA), contaminated salmon in, 78
San Francisco Bay (CA), mercury in, 6
Sanita Pubblica, 130, 139
sardines
  anisakid nematodes and, 145
  dioxins in, 141
  marine algae and, 89
  PAHs in, 23, 137
  parasites in, 38

PCBs/PCDFs in, 10
  scromboid food poisoning and, 19
sarpa salpa, hallucinogenic poison from, 102
Sauvé, Sébastien, 43
Savannah River Basin, PCBs in, 53
saxitoxin, Florida advisory about, 12
schizophrenia, omega-3 fatty acids and, 58
Science, 78, 92
Science Daily, 60, 62
Science News, 101, 102
Science of the Total Environment, 132, 133, 135, 140
scientists' recommendations, about oceans' health, 104
scombroid poisoning, 19, 147
Scotland, 78, 101
sea bass, 131
seafood. *See also* specific types of
  BMAA in, 27
  dioxins in, 141
  metals in, 141–42
  PCBs in, 27, 140
  in Singaporean study, 140
sea level, rising of, 97
sea vegetables, 108, 109
Second Opinion, 68
Seeliger, Bruce, 34
selective serotonin reuptake inhibitors (SSRIs), as endocrine disruptors, 54–55
selenium, in US freshwater fish, 136
sensory-motor problems, mercury and, 34
sertraline, as endocrine disruptor, 55
sesame seeds, as omega-3 fatty acid source, 71
17alpha-ethinylestradiol (EE2), 146
17beta-estradiol, 50, 51
sewage, in deep seas, 98, 99, 104
sexual changes, 41–42, 46, 50
sexual intercourse, ciguatera poisoning and, 19
shampoo chemicals, as endocrine disruptors, 50
Shannon International River Basin District (Ireland), 46
sharks, 6, 7, 13, 131
shellfish
  BMAA in, 27
  dioxins in, 140
  farm-raised, 88
  food poisoning and, 18, 19
  mercury in, 131, 133
  PBDEs in, 27
  PCBs in, 130, 139
shrimp. *See also* specific types of
  biomagnification and, 13
  omega-3 fatty acids in, 131
  PAHs and, 11
  PAHs in, 23, 137
Sierra Nevada Mountains, mercury contamination and, 6
Singaporean seafood studies, 10, 27, 140
skinned fish, contaminants "reduced" by, 36, 81
smallmouth bass, 11, 42, 54
smoked fish/meat
  cancer and, 129

About the Author

Brian Clement, PhD, NMD, LN, has spent more than four decades researching and practicing nutrition and progressive health care. He has graduate degrees in both naturopathic medicine and nutritional science. He has guided the Hippocrates Health Institute in West Palm Beach, Florida, since 1980.

In his role as an educator, Dr. Clement has conducted countless seminars, lectures, and educational programs in more than forty countries. His ideas on natural health, along with his vast theoretical and practical scientific experience, have earned him a reputation as a leading expert in advancing the fields of preventive medicine and natural health. He has been commissioned by government-supported organizations to establish, organize, and direct health programs in Denmark, Ireland, Switzerland, Greece, and India.

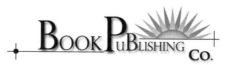

BOOK PUBLISHING CO.

books that educate, inspire, and empower
To find your favorite vegetarian and soyfood products online, visit:
www.healthy-eating.com

More titles by
Brian R. Clement

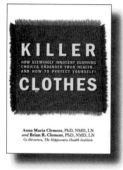

Killer Chlothes
How Seemingly Innocent Clothing
Choices Endanger Your Health …
and How to Protect Yourself!
978-1-57067-263-7 $14.95

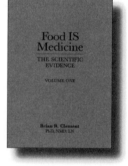

Food IS Medicine
The Scientific Evidence
978-1-57067-274-3 $29.95

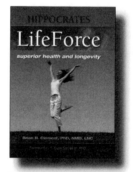

Hippocrates LifeForce
Superior Health and Longevity
978-1-57067-249-1 $14.95

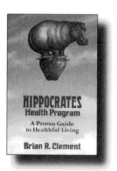

Hippocrates Health Program
A Proven Guide to Healthful Living
978-0-9622373-0-0 $7.95

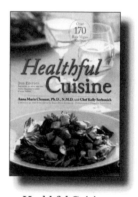

Healthful Cuisine
2nd Edition
978-1-57067-175-3 $17.95

Purchase these health titles and cookbooks from your local bookstore or natural food store,
or you can buy them directly from:

Book Publishing Company • P.O. Box 99 • Summertown, TN 38483 • 1-800-695-2241

Please include $3.95 per book for shipping and handling.